THE
BIG BOOK
OF BIBLE
CURES

VOLUME 1: WEIGHT LOSS

THE
BIG BOOK
OF BIBLE
CURES

VOLUME 1: WEIGHT LOSS

DON COLBERT, MD

SILOAM

Most CHARISMA HOUSE BOOK GROUP products are available at special quantity discounts for bulk purchase for sales promotions, premiums, fundraising, and educational needs. For details, write Charisma House Book Group, 600 Rinehart Road, Lake Mary, Florida 32746, or telephone (407) 333-0600.

THE BIG BOOK OF BIBLE CURES VOLUME 1: WEIGHT LOSS
  by Don Colbert, MD
Published by Siloam
Charisma Media/Charisma House Book Group
600 Rinehart Road
Lake Mary, Florida 32746
www.charismahouse.com

Scripture quotations marked KJV are from the King James Version of the Bible.

Scripture quotations marked NASB are from the New American Standard Bible, copyright © 1960, 1962, 1963, 1968, 1971, 1972, 1973, 1975, 1977, 1995 by The Lockman Foundation. Used by permission. (www.Lockman.org)

Scripture quotations marked NKJV are taken from the New King James Version®. Copyright © 1982 by Thomas Nelson. Used by permission. All rights reserved.

Scripture quotations marked NLT are from the Holy Bible, New Living Translation, copyright © 1996, 2004, 2007. Used by permission of Tyndale House Publishers, Inc., Wheaton, IL 60189. All rights reserved.

Cover design by Justin Evans

The New Bible Cure for Weight Loss was previously published separately by Siloam, ISBN 987-1-61638-616-0, copyright © 2013.

The Bible Cure for Thyroid Disorders was previously published separately by Siloam, ISBN 978-1-59185-281-0, copyright © 2004.

The New Bible Cure for Diabetes was previously published separately by Siloam, ISBN 978-1-59979-759-5, copyright © 2009.

The Bible Cure for Candida and Yeast Infections was previously published separately by Siloam, ISBN 978-0-88419-743-0, copyright © 2001.

The Bible Cure for Recipes for Overcoming Candida was previously published separately by Siloam, ISBN 978-0-88419-940-3, copyright © 2004.

International Standard Book Number: 978-1-62998-949-5

E-book ISBN: 978-1-62998-950-1

17 18 19 20 21 — 9 8 7 6 5 4 3 2 1

Printed in the United States of America

CONTENTS

The New Bible Cure for Weight Loss

The Bible Cure for Thyroid Disorders

The New Bible Cure for Diabetes

The Bible Cure for Candida and Yeast Infections

The Bible Cure Recipes for Overcoming Candida

THE NEW BIBLE
CURE
FOR WEIGHT LOSS

Chapter 1

YOU ARE GOD'S MASTERPIECE!

BEFORE THE FINGER of God touched the oceans with unimaginable creative power, God envisioned you in His heart. He saw you and all you could be one day through the power of His supernatural grace.

You are God's masterpiece, designed according to an eternal plan so awesome that it's beyond your ability to comprehend. Have you ever wondered what He saw in His mind when He created you? What was the perfection of purpose and plan He intended?

Now close your eyes and see yourself. For one moment you have no bondages, no imperfections, no shortcomings. Your body is as lean and healthy as it could possibly be. What do you look like? Is that the person God had in mind?

If you've struggled with obesity all of your life, you may not even be able to imagine yourself free of the bondage of unwanted fat. But God can. Don't you think that if God is powerful enough to create you and the entire universe that you see around you, He is also able to help you overcome all of your personal bondages? Of course He is!

That's what this Bible Cure is all about. It is a plan of godly principles, wisdom, and scriptural advice to help deliver you from an unhealthy lifestyle and future ill health and to give you the freedom and joy of a healthy, fit, more attractive you!

AN OBESITY EPIDEMIC

If you have a weight problem, you're not alone. The terms *overweight* and *obese* are defined using the body mass index (BMI), which evaluates a person's weight relative to height. Various health organizations, including the Centers for Disease Control and Prevention (CDC) and the National Institutes of Health (NIH), define an overweight adult as having a BMI between 25 and 29.9, while an obese adult is anyone with a BMI of 30 or higher.[1]

In the last several years America has experienced an alarming arise in obesity. Two-thirds of American adults are overweight or obese, and 30 percent of children age eleven or younger are overweight.[2] This should concern everyone, particularly those of us who professes Jesus as Savior and Lord. God revealed His divine will for each of us through the apostle John, who wrote, "Beloved, I pray that you may prosper in all things and be in health, just as your soul prospers" (3 John 2, NKJV). With obesity at almost epidemic proportions, surely we are missing God's best.

A DEADLY KILLER

Research tells us that, in the United States, an estimated 300,000 deaths per year are attributed to obesity.[3] Obesity also comes with a fat price tag (pun intended). People considered obese pay $1,429 more (42 percent) in health care costs than normal weight individuals.[4] And as shocking as all this sounds, no dollar amount can do justice to the real damage being done. Being overweight or obese increases your risk of developing thirty-five major diseases, particularly type 2 diabetes, heart disease, stroke, arthritis, hypertension, acid reflux, sleep apnea, Alzheimer's, infertility, erectile dysfunction, and gallbladder disease— plus more than a dozen forms of cancer.

Besides obesity's physical implications, it carries a social and psychological impact. Obese individuals generally contend with more rejection and prejudice. Often they are overlooked for promotions or not even hired because of physical appearance. Most obese people struggle daily with issues of self-worth and self-image. They feel unattractive and unappreciated and are at an increased risk of depression. Many of us have watched the humiliation an obese person experiences trying to squeeze into an airplane, stadium, or automobile seat that is too small. Maybe you have been that person. If so, you know how obesity can affect the way others treat you and how you treat yourself.

POWER FOR SUCCESS

Instead of looking for the next new-and-improved medication to manage obesity-related disease, we need to get to the root of the problem, which is our diet, lifestyle, and waistline. The standard American diet is full of empty carbohydrates, sugars, fats, excessive proteins, and calories, and it is low in nutrient content. Combined with our poor diet is a lack of physical activity and excessive stress that usually raises cortisol levels. Because of this increase of cortisol, many are developing toxic belly fat, which increases their risk for incurring a host of other diseases, including diabetes.

This simple Bible Cure provides all you need for health and successful weight loss to help you become the person you saw or imagined when you closed your eyes. With fresh understanding, proper nutrition, exercise, and supplements you can find all the physical elements you need for radical change. Mixed together with the power of God found in prayer and Scripture, you will discover strength for success that is beyond your own ability.

Originally published as *The Bible Cure for Weight Loss and Muscle Gain* in 2000, *The New Bible Cure for Weight Loss* has been revised and updated with the latest medical research on ways to reduce your waistline, control your weight, and rid yourself of the toxic body fat that leads to so many diseases. If you compare it side by side with the previous edition, you'll see that it's also larger, allowing me to expand greatly upon the information provided in the previous edition and provide you with a deeper understanding of what you face and how to overcome it.

Unchanged from the previous edition are the timeless, life-changing, and healing scriptures throughout this book that will strengthen and encourage your spirit and soul. The proven principles, truths, and guidelines in these passages anchor the practical and medical insights also contained in this book. They will effectively focus your prayers, thoughts, and actions so you can step into God's plan of divine health for you—a plan that includes victory over obesity.

Another change since the original *The Bible Cure for Weight Loss and Muscle Gain* was published is that I've released two important books on weight loss, *The Rapid Waist Reduction Diet* and *Dr. Colbert's "I Can Do This" Diet.* I encourage you to read those books, because they delve even deeper into the changes that will empower you to lose weight and keep it off. I also recommend my book *The Seven Pillars of Health* because the principles it contains are the foundation to healthy living that will affect all areas of your life. It sets the stage for everything you will ever read in any other book I've published—including this one.

I pray that these spiritual and practical suggestions for health, nutrition, and fitness will bring wholeness to your life, increase your spiritual understanding, and strengthen your ability to worship and serve God.

There is much you can do to change the course of your health. As you learn about obesity, understand its causes, and take the practical, positive steps detailed in this book, you will defeat obesity in your life and discover the abundant life promised by Jesus when He said, "I have come that they may have life, and that they may have it more abundantly" (John 10:10, NKJV).

Now is the time to run to the battle with fresh confidence, renewed determination, and the wonderful knowledge that God is real, alive, and more powerful than any sickness or disease. It is my prayer that my suggestions and guidelines will help improve your health, nutritional habits, and fitness practices. This combination will bring wholeness to your life. I pray that they will deepen your fellowship with God and strengthen your ability to worship and serve Him.

A **BIBLE CURE** *Prayer for You*

I pray that God will fill you with hope, encouragement, and wisdom as you read this book. May He give you the willpower to make healthy choices about your nutrition, exercise, and lifestyle. May He strengthen your resolve to maintain a healthy weight and not to overtax your body with excessive weight. I pray that you live a long and prosperous life living in divine health so that you may fulfill your purpose and serve the Lord. Amen.

Chapter 2

DID YOU KNOW?—
UNDERSTANDING OBESITY

THE BIBLE INSTRUCTS us to be wise in our eating habits: "Whether you eat or drink, or whatever you do, do all to the glory of God" (1 Cor. 10:31, NKJV). The way you eat, drink, and care for the body that God gave you can bring glory to Him for this wonderful gift.

Chances are that if you are struggling with obesity, you may have been waging a war with it all of your life. By now you realize that you need more than a good dieting program. You need power to enforce it. You need the strength it takes to change a lifetime of poor eating habits and the discipline to stay with it. This Bible Cure pathway to wholeness not only provides the information necessary for a healthier, trimmer body, but it also provides insight into an endless source of power to insure success. Stop limiting yourself to your own strength. The Bible reveals a better way:

> I can do all things through Christ who strengthens me.
> —PHILIPPIANS 4:13, NKJV

Gaining new power in your battle against obesity must begin with gaining fresh understanding of the causes for obesity.

WHY WE EAT TOO MUCH

Being overweight has many causes. Some are biological. You might be predisposed to obesity through genetics and body metabolism. Some of the causes are psychological.

5

Emotional eating

You also may be emotionally dependent on food for comfort during times of stress, crisis, anxiety, loneliness, and a host of other emotions. If overeating has an emotional component in your life, you probably grew up hearing statements such as the following:

- "Eat something; it will make you feel better."
- "Clean your plate, or you can't leave the table."
- "If you're good, you will get dessert."
- "If you don't eat everything, you will be impolite to the host or hostess."
- "If you stop crying, I'll give you ice cream."

> Through the LORD's mercies we are not consumed, because His compassions fail not. They are new every morning; great is Your faithfulness.
> —LAMENTATIONS 3:22–23, NKJV

The list of unhealthy childhood motivations can be endless. But whether the causes of your weight problem are genetic or psychological, you are not bound to your past. Today is a new day, filled with fresh hope for an entirely new way of thinking and living. Begin considering what lifestyle factors might be contributing to your situation.

A sedentary lifestyle

Another cause of obesity is the increasingly sedentary lifestyle in our society. In an agricultural or industrial culture hard work gives people plenty of exercise during the day. In our corporate, technological culture we sit more at desks and in meetings. What about you? The problem doesn't just plague adults. Too many children no longer play sports and participate in outdoor activities. Instead they get entranced by video games, smartphones, text messages, social networking, online media, TV, and movies. Combined with their favorite fast food, reducing exercise to a flick of the finger on a remote control spells ever-increasing weight gain.

Excessive stress

The excessive stress that most adults and many children labor under also contributes to our expanding waistlines. Stress increases cortisol levels. As a result, many are developing toxic belly fat, thereby increasing their risk for incurring diabetes and other diseases. Long-term stress eventually depletes stress hormones as well as neurotransmitters. This often helps unleash ravenous appetites, plus addictions to sugar and carbohydrates. It's like a nightmarish vortex, each bad habit working to ensnare sufferers in a downward spiral to poor health and disease.

Too much refined sugar and starch

I believe one of the most important reasons for our epidemic of obesity is our high intake of both refined sugars and starches. The standard American diet is full of empty carbohydrates, sugars, fats, excessive proteins, and calories, and it is low in nutrient content. This diet literally causes us to lose nutrients such as chromium, which is crucial in regulating glucose levels in our blood.

The average person consumes 130 pounds of refined sugar per year.[1] These sugars are sometimes hidden in foods we think are good for us. Take a look at how most of our bread is made. First the outer shell of the grain of wheat is removed. This is the bran or the fiber portion of the grain. The germ of the wheat is then removed; the germ contains the essential fats and vitamin E. These are removed to affect the shelf life of the bread. What is left over is the endosperm, which is the starch of the grain. This is then ground into a very fine powder. The powder of the grain, however, is not white, so it is then bleached with a bleaching agent.

With both the bran and the wheat germ no longer present, and after the bleaching process, very few vitamins remain. Therefore man-made vitamins are then added back, along with sugar, salt, partially hydrogenated fats, and preservatives. White bread is very constipating because it contains no fiber. Also, since it is highly processed when it is consumed, it is rapidly broken down into sugars, and this then causes high amounts of insulin to be secreted, putting a strain on the pancreas and programming our body to store fat.

I believe that increased consumption of white bread, sugar,

processed cereals, and pasta is largely responsible for our epidemic of diabetes, high cholesterol, heart disease, and obesity. In centuries past, these refined breads and sugars were given mainly to extremely rich and royal families. This is why many of the wealthy in those days were obese and suffered from diabetes and gout.

A Word About Wheat

The problem with breads, pastas, cereals, and other starches may not be limited to the refining process they undergo. The wheat itself may be the real culprit. Renowned cardiologist William Davis, MD, believes foods made with or containing wheat are the number one reason Americans are fat and suffering from diabetes. Modern wheat strains have been hybridized, crossbred, and genetically altered by agricultural scientists in order to increase crop production.[2] As a result, modern strains of wheat have a "higher quantity of genes for gluten proteins that are associated with celiac disease."[3] Modern wheat also contains a starch called amylopectin A, which raises blood sugar levels more than virtually any other carbohydrate.[4]

In addition, wheat is an appetite stimulant, making you want more and more food.[5] It's also considered addictive. Approximately 30 percent of all people who stop eating wheat products experience withdrawal symptoms such as extreme fatigue, mental fog, irritability, inability to function at work, and depression.[6] The addictive nature of wheat, coupled with the fact that it triggers exaggerated blood sugar and insulin responses, sets your body up to pack on the pounds.

Sugar and Your Body

A lot of people think eating fat makes you fat. It's actually the way your body stores fat that makes you gain weight. Overconsumption of carbohydrates and sugars stimulates your body's production of insulin—which is the body's fat storage hormone. Insulin lowers blood sugar levels when they are too high. However, elevated insulin levels also cause the body to store fat.

For example, when you eat foods that are high in carbohydrates, such as breads, pasta, potatoes, corn, and rice, the carbohydrate is broken down to glucose, which is absorbed into the bloodstream. If insulin levels are elevated, the carbohydrate is more likely to be converted to fat by the liver and then stored away in fat cells.

Easier On Than Off

If you consume a lot of starch and sugar on a frequent basis, your insulin levels will remain high. If insulin levels remain high, your fat is, figuratively speaking, locked into your fat cells. This makes it very easy to gain weight and extremely difficult to lose weight. Elevated insulin levels usually prevent the body from burning stored body fat for energy. Most obese patients cannot break out of this vicious cycle because they are constantly craving starchy, sugary foods throughout the day, which keeps the insulin levels elevated and prevents the body from burning these stored fats.

> Hear me, O LORD, for Your lovingkindness is good; turn to me according to the multitude of Your tender mercies. And do not hide Your face from Your servant, for I am in trouble; hear me speedily.
> —PSALM 69:16–17, NKJV

The average person can store about 300–400 grams of carbohydrates in the muscles and about 90 grams in the liver. The stored carbohydrates are actually a stored form of glucose called glycogen. However, once the body storehouses are filled in the liver and muscles, any excess carbohydrates are then usually converted into fat and stored in fatty tissues. When one skips meals or goes over four to five hours without eating, the blood sugar usually decreases, unleashing a ravenous appetite.

Exercise may not help you if you don't eat right. If you eat refined carbohydrates throughout the day, much of the excess carbohydrates will be converted to fat. The high insulin levels also make it more difficult for the body not to release a significant amount of its stored fat. Therefore you can work out for hours at a gym and still not lose fat because you are eating high amounts of carbohydrates and sugar throughout the day. Your body usually will store excess carbohydrates as fat and make it difficult to release any fat that is already stored.

To make matters even worse, when you consume sugar or starches frequently, especially cake, candy, cookies, fruit juices, ice cream, or processed white flour, you may develop low blood sugar within a few hours after eating and unleash a ravenous appetite for more sugar and starch. This raises your blood sugar and your insulin levels, programming you for even more fat storage and preventing you from burning stored fat when you exercise. How frustrating this can be for the uninformed patient. Symptoms of low blood sugar include spaciness, shakiness, irritability, extreme fatigue, headache, sweatiness, racing heart, extreme hunger, or an extreme craving for sweets or starches.

CAUGHT IN A TRAP

This creates a vicious cycle. If you don't eat something sweet or starchy every few hours, you may develop the symptoms of low blood sugar. This is a very important point. You can turn this entire situation around very easily by taking a very simple step: *avoid sugar and refined starches.*

By avoiding sweets, starches, snack foods, junk foods, or high-carbohydrate foods, you can lower your insulin levels and turn off the main trigger that is telling the body to store fat and preventing the body from releasing fat.

When the brain doesn't get enough glucose, you will get cravings. The brain requires a constant supply of glucose. When too much insulin is secreted, such as when you consume a snack that is high in sugar (i.e., a doughnut, a Coke, or cookies), the pancreas then responds by secreting enough insulin to lower the sugar. Often too much insulin is secreted, which lowers the sugar too much, thus causing low blood sugar. Since the brain is not getting the glucose it requires, the low blood sugar creates sugar and carbohydrate cravings, extreme hunger, mood swings, fatigue, and problems concentrating. The brain releases different hormones to increase one's appetite. These signals cause the individual to reach for a sugar or starch "fix" in order to raise the blood sugar the fastest, which will then be able to supply the brain with adequate glucose.

THE POWER OF GLUCAGON

Glucagon is a hormone that works totally opposite than insulin works. Insulin is a fat-storing hormone, whereas glucagon is a fat-releasing hormone. In other words, glucagon will actually enable the body to release stored body fat from the fatty tissues and will permit your muscle tissues to burn your fat as the preferred fuel source instead of blood sugar.

How do you release this powerful substance into your body? It's easy. The release of glucagon is stimulated by eating a correct amount of protein in a meal along with the proper balance of fats and carbohydrates. We will look at this in greater detail later on.

> My flesh and my heart fail; but God is the strength of my heart and my portion forever.
> —PSALM 73:26, NKJV

When the insulin levels are high in the body, the level of glucagon is low. When glucagon is high, then insulin is low. When you eat a lot of sugar and starch, you raise your insulin levels and lower your glucagon, thus preventing fat from being released to be used as fuel. By simply stabilizing your blood sugar and lowering your insulin levels, you can keep your glucagon levels elevated, which enables your body to burn off the extra fat. Thus you'll begin to realize a more energetic, slimmer you! Eating your protein first helps boost glucagon levels, or you can eat a salad with sliced chicken, turkey, or fish.

SHOULD YOU COUNT CALORIES?

Many people still say, "Why not count calories? A calorie is a calorie." Most people believe that since fat has 9 calories per gram and carbohydrates have only 4 calories per gram, then eating a gram of fat is much more fattening than eating a gram of carbohydrate. But the hormonal effects of fat are not nearly as dramatic as the hormonal effects of carbohydrates and sugars.

Fats will not raise insulin levels, which programs the body to store fat. However, sugars and starches will trigger dramatic releases of insulin, which is the most powerful fat-storing hormone. So don't count calories. Instead, be aware of how your body works. Keep in mind the powerful hormonal effects that sugars and starches have on both insulin, the fat-storing hormone, and on glucagon, the fat-releasing hormone.

The Bible says, "Surely, in vain the net is spread in the sight of any bird" (Prov. 1:17, NKJV). That means you cannot capture a prey if it understands what's happening. By understanding this powerful truth about how your body actually works, you can avoid the trap of high blood sugar, of high insulin levels, of being overweight or obese, and even of diabetes. Now that you know, the power is in your hands!

GLYCEMIC INDEX 101

The glycemic index was created in the early 1980s to track how quickly insulin levels shot up in individuals after they consumed carbohydrates. While studying individuals with type 2 diabetes, researchers found that certain carbohydrates increased blood sugar levels and insulin levels, while other carbohydrates did not.

They tested hundreds of different foods to determine their glycemic index value. Because their methods and findings have proven so reliable, they are the standard by which we measure the internal processing of foods.

The glycemic index assigns a numeric value to how rapidly the blood sugar rises after consuming a food that contains carbohydrates. Sugars and carbohydrates that are digested rapidly, such as white bread, white rice, and instant potatoes, rapidly increase blood sugar. These are high-glycemic foods and have a glycemic index of 70 or higher. On the other hand, if foods containing carbohydrates are digested slowly and therefore release sugars gradually into the bloodstream, they have a glycemic index value of 55 or lower. These foods include most vegetables and fruits, beans, peas, lentils, sweet potatoes, and the like.

Because these foods cause the blood sugar to rise more slowly, blood sugar levels are stabilized for a longer period of time. Low-glycemic foods also cause satiety hormones to be released in the small intestines, which satisfies you for longer periods of time.

A **BIBLE CURE** *Health Fact*

Rule of Thumb: The Glycemic Index

Low-glycemic foods: 55 or less
Medium-glycemic foods: 56 to 69
High-glycemic foods: 70 or above

In truth, there is nothing fancy about the glycemic index. The degree to which a food has been processed is one of the most important factors that determine its glycemic index value. Generally speaking, the more highly a food is processed, the higher its glycemic index value; the more natural a food, the lower its value.

THE GLYCEMIC LOAD

Almost twenty years after the glycemic index was created, researchers at Harvard University developed a new way of classifying foods that took into account not only the glycemic index value of a food but also the quantity of carbohydrates that particular food contains. This is called the glycemic load (GL). It serves as a guide as to how much of a particular carbohydrate or food we should eat.

For a while nutritionists scratched their heads over patients who wanted to lose weight and were eating low-glycemic foods yet weren't shedding many pounds. Some actually gained weight. Through the GL they discovered that overconsuming many low-glycemic foods can actually lead to weight gain. Not surprisingly, many patients were eating as many low-glycemic foods as they wanted, simply because they had been told that foods with a low value promoted weight loss. They needed to know the whole story, which is how the glycemic load balanced the picture. A food's GL is determined by multiplying the glycemic index value by the quantity of carbohydrates a serving contains (in grams), and then dividing that number by 100. The actual formula looks like this:

- (Glycemic Index Value x Carb Grams per Serving) ÷ 100 = Glycemic Load

To show you how important the GL is, let me offer some examples. Some wheat pastas have a low glycemic index value, which makes many dieters think they're automatically a key to losing weight. However, if a serving size of that wheat pasta is too large, it may sabotage your weight-loss efforts. Despite a low glycemic index value, the pasta's GL is high. Another example is white potatoes, which have a GL double that of yams. On the other end of the scale, watermelon has a high glycemic index value but a very low GL, which makes it OK to eat in a larger quantity.

Don't worry, though. You will not have to calculate the GL for every item you eat. By understanding the GL, you can identify which low-glycemic foods can cause trouble if you eat too much of them. These include low-glycemic breads, low-glycemic rice, sweet potatoes, yams, low-glycemic pasta, low-glycemic cereals, and so forth. As a general rule, any large quantity of a low-glycemic "starchy" food will usually have a high GL.

GLYCEMIC INDEX VALUES OF COMMON FOODS[7]			
Food*	Glycemic Index Value	Food	Glycemic Index Value
Asparagus	15	Broccoli	15
Celery	15	Cucumber	15
Green beans	15	Low-fat yogurt (artificially sweetened)	15
Peppers (all varieties)	15	Spinach	15
Zucchini	15	Tomatoes	15
Cherries	22	Green peas	22
Black beans	30	Milk (skim)	32
Apples	36	Spaghetti (whole wheat)	37
All-Bran cereal	42	Lentil soup (canned)	44

GLYCEMIC INDEX VALUES OF COMMON FOODS[7]			
Food*	Glycemic Index Value	Food	Glycemic Index Value
Orange juice	52	Bananas	53
Potato (sweet)	54	Rice (brown)	55
Popcorn	55	Muesli	56
Whole-wheat bread	69	Watermelon	72
Doughnut	75	Rice cakes	82
Corn flakes	84	Potato (baked)	85
Baguette (French bread)	95	Parsnips	97

* To look up the glycemic index values of other foods not listed above, go to www.thecandodiet.com or http://tinyurl.com/glycemic-index-list.

The amount of fiber in your food, the amount of fat, how much sugar is in the carbohydrates, and proteins all determine the glycemic index score of what you eat.

THREE TYPES OF SUGAR

Three main types of simple sugars (called monosaccharides) make up all carbohydrates. These include:

- Glucose
- Fructose
- Galactose

Glucose is found in breads, cereals, starches, pasta, and grains. Fructose is found in fruits, and galactose is found in dairy products. Plain sugar, or sucrose, is a disaccharide and consists of glucose and fructose joined.

The liver rapidly absorbs these simple sugars. However, only glucose can be released directly back into the bloodstream. Fructose and galactose must first be converted to glucose in the liver to gain entrance into the bloodstream. Thus they are released at a much slower rate. Fructose, found primarily in fruits, has a low glycemic index compared to glucose and galactose.

OTHER GLYCEMIC FOODS

Fiber is a form of carbohydrate that is not absorbed. However, it does slow down the rate of absorption of other carbohydrates. Thus the higher the fiber content of the carbohydrate or starch, the more slowly it will be absorbed and enter the bloodstream. Most fruits are high in fiber and have a low glycemic value. The exceptions are bananas, raisins, dates, and other dried fruits. Almost all vegetables are high in fiber and low-glycemic except for potatoes, carrots, corn, and beets, which have a high glycemic value.

In the next chapter we will discuss in more detail the best foods to eat for overall good health and especially if you want to lose weight. The right carbohydrates balanced with the proper portions of proteins and fats will create a much lower glycemic effect on your body and interrupt the vicious cycle of weight gain.

> I will be glad and rejoice in Your mercy, for You have considered my trouble; You have known my soul in adversities.
> —PSALM 31:7, NKJV

THE WORST KIND OF FAT

You may not like the number on your scale, but that figure does not tell the whole story regarding your overall health. Researchers are finding that one of the greatest indicators of potential health problems is having a high percentage of belly fat. The fat that settles in the belly is different from other types of fat in the body. Fatty tissue or fat storage areas, such as belly fat, are active endocrine organs that produce numerous types of hormones, such as resistin (which increases insulin resistance), leptin (which decreases appetite), and adiponectin (which improves insulin sensitivity and helps to lower blood sugar). The more belly fat cells you have, typically the more estrogen, cortisol, and testosterone your body produces. This is one of the reasons obese men typically develop breasts and obese women often grow hair on their faces. Their fat cells are manufacturing more estrogen and testosterone, respectively.

When your fatty tissues spew out all these hormones—most likely raising your estrogen, testosterone, and cortisol levels—and produce tremendous inflammation in your body, the result is weight gain. Your extra toxic belly fat then sets the stage for type 2 diabetes, heart disease, stroke, cancer, and a host of other diseases. That's because belly fat is like a wildfire. It spreads throughout your body and inflames your cardiovascular system, which eventually causes the production of plaque in your arteries and inflammation in the brain. This can even potentially lead to Alzheimer's disease.

The dangers of this toxic belly fat is one reason this Bible Cure encourages you to set a weight-loss goal based on your waistline rather than your body weight. Typically if your waist measurement increases, your blood sugar will increase; if your waist measurement decreases, your blood sugar will decrease. By reducing your waist measurement, you will probably reverse your risk of many diseases. In fact, lowering waist size ranks higher than weight loss.

Although it is helpful to weigh yourself on a regular basis, I want you to start looking at your waistline as a key indicator of weight management. You should measure your waist around your navel (and love handles, if you have them). Initially your waist measurement goal should be 40 inches or less if you're a man and 35 inches or less if you're a woman. But your ultimate goal should be to have a waist measurement that is half your height or less. For example, a 5-foot-10-inch man is 70 inches tall, so his waist around the belly button and love handles should be 35 inches or less.

OTHER WEIGHT MANAGEMENT MEASURES

While I see waist size as the most important measurement for establishing weight-loss goals, another key measurement is body fat percentage. There are many ways to measure body fat percentage, including a bioimpedance analysis, underwater weighing, and using skinfold calipers. Whatever the method, you need to have your body fat percentage measured the same way each time. Consistency is the key, since the percentage can fluctuate dramatically with inaccurate measurements.

I hold more stock in body fat percentage than I do the body mass index reading. The reason is simple: accuracy. BMI uses only height and weight to judge how overweight or obese a person is. For example, a twenty-three-year-old professional football player and a fifty-six-year-old executive may both be 5 feet 10 inches tall and weigh 220 pounds. This gives both men a BMI of approximately 35, which is considered obese.

In reality, however, the football player can have a 32-inch waist and a remarkable 6 percent body fat; the executive can have a 44-inch waist and 33 percent body fat. That is an astounding 27 percent differential in body fat percentage alone, which the BMI doesn't take into account.

Although many physicians simply use BMI to determine if a person is overweight or obese, I strongly believe more accurate assessments come from using body fat percentage and waist measurements. However, because it is a helpful tool to measure your weight loss goals, I have included the following chart to help you determine your BMI.

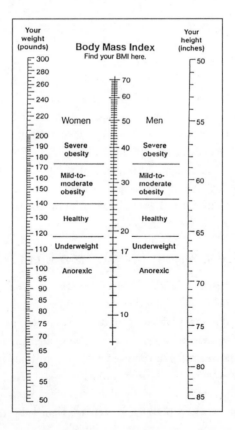

RATING YOUR BODY FAT PERCENTAGE

According to the American Council on Exercise, a body fat percentage greater than 25 percent in men and greater than 33 percent in women is considered obese. A healthy percent body fat in women is 25–31 percent and in men is 18–25 percent.[8]

Initially, obese men should aim for a reading of less than 25 percent, while obese women should shoot for less than 33 percent. Eventually aim for a percent body fat in the healthy range. However, body fat ranks second to your initial focus to reduce your waist measurement.

Many health clubs, nutritionists, and physicians have the equipment to measure your percentage of body fat. Once you have this initial number, monitor it each month.

However, don't get too hung up on body fat or other measurements like your BMI reading. Mainly focus on one thing and one thing only: your waist measurement. You really do not need a scale or any other fancy tools—just a tape measure. By focusing on your waist and achieving your goal measurement, you will eliminate one of the main risk factors for disease.

> His divine power has given to us all things that pertain to life and godliness, through the knowledge of Him who called us by glory and virtue.
>
> —2 PETER 1:3, NKJV

If you see yourself in the symptoms I've described in this chapter, don't wait. Make a decision to stop the process of disease in your body right now. God will help you to stay with it if you give Him an opportunity. Why not turn this entire matter over to Him right now? God is at your side to help you. He promises, "I will never leave you nor forsake you" (Heb. 13:5, NKJV). God is your helper and loves you more than you will ever know. He longs to give you all the strength, power, and hope you need to triumph in your battle. Pray this Bible Cure prayer and keep pressing forward.

A **BIBLE CURE** *Prayer for You*

Lord God, You alone are my strength and my source. My ability to stay committed to weight loss and healthy eating comes from You. Help me to maintain the willpower I need to eliminate sugar and empty calories from my diet. Give me the focus I need to implement all that I am learning. Almighty God, replace any discouragement with hope and any doubt with faith. I know that You are with me and will not leave me. I thank You, Lord, for seeing me through this battle and giving me victory over obesity. Amen.

R℞

A **BIBLE CURE** *Prescription*

Measure your waistline at your navel; write down the figure:

_____

Write down your goal waist measurement: _____

Take a brief self-assessment by answering the following questions.

❏ How many times a day do you eat sugars and carbohydrates?

_____

_____

❏ Describe how you can reduce that frequency.

_____

_____

❏ List the foods high in sugar and starch that you need to eliminate from your diet:

_____

_____

_____

❏ What foods high in protein and fiber can you add to your diet? What high-glycemic foods can you eliminate?

_____

_____

_____

Chapter 3

THE FOUNDATION OF HEALTHY EATING

G OD SKILLFULLY DESIGNED your body as an incredible, living creation that will operate at peak efficiency and health when it is supplied with proper nutrition. In the previous chapter we looked at many of the reasons Americans are obese. Now I want to take a look at the powerful nutritional foundation that will help you to discover a healthier, happier, more attractive you.

CHOOSING THE RIGHT CARBOHYDRATES

Certain carbohydrates are critical for good health. When combined with the correct portions of fats and proteins, good carbs give you energy, calm your mood, keep you full and satisfied by turning off hunger, and assist in weight loss. They also help you to enjoy meals and snacks, enable you to handle stress better, allow you to sleep more soundly, improve your bowel function, and give you an overall feeling of well-being.

However, as with so many things in the land of excess, most Americans have fallen in love with the wrong kind of carbs. They see their waistlines getting wider and wider as a result of eating too much sugar, starch, bread, and pasta, and think the answer is to swear off all carbohydrates. The problem is, high-protein diets are often hard to maintain for long and in some cases they have damaging effects on health. The answer isn't a no-carb diet, but one rich in the right kinds of carbohydrates.

The National Institutes of Health recommends that 45 to 65 percent of daily energy intake for adults come from carbohydrates, with 20 to 35 percent of energy coming from fats, and only 10 to 35 percent from proteins.[1] The American Diabetes Association also recommends

45 to 60 grams of carbohydrates in each meal, preferably from healthy whole grains. I believe this is too many carbohydrates and too much grain. I believe excessive carbohydrates and grains—especially wheat and corn products—are one of the main reasons for our obesity epidemic. I typically recommend about 50 to 55 percent of daily calories come from low-glycemic carbohydrates, 15 to 20 percent from plant and lean animal proteins, and 25 to 30 percent from healthy fats.

Because wheat and corn can trigger exaggerated blood sugar responses, I have my patients give up all wheat and corn products for a season or until they reduce their belly or body fat. Even if breads at the supermarket are called whole-grain breads, they still contain amylopectin A, which usually spikes blood sugar, programming the body for fat storage and weight gain. Therefore if my patients request bread, I recommend that they have small amounts of millet bread in the morning or at lunch. It contains no wheat. However, if weight loss stalls, I have my patients stop eating millet bread. Once a person reaches his goal waist measurement or weight, if he can practice moderation, I have him add back small servings of wheat and corn for breakfast or lunch, but not dinner.

The Tortoise and the Hare

So how can a person know which are the right carbs to choose? Many people are familiar with the old story about the tortoise and the hare. The hare races ahead but fails to reach the finish line, while the slow but steady tortoise eventually passes him and wins the race. When it comes to how your body processes carbohydrates, the race that takes place within you is reminiscent of this classic fable. I've used these familiar characters to identify two main types of carbohydrates we will talk about in this Bible Cure: low-glycemic "tortoise carbs" and high-glycemic "hare carbs."

> I will love You, O LORD, my strength.
>
> —PSALM 18:1, NKJV

Unfortunately most of the carbohydrates overweight and obese people consume are high-glycemic "hare carbs," which cause the blood sugar to rise rapidly. As I have already alluded to, this starts a chain of events that trap people in a fat-storage mode and prevent them from losing weight. The underlying cycle of hare carbs is obvious enough: the faster you absorb the carbs, the higher your insulin level rises, the more weight you gain, and the more diseases you develop. You become literally programmed for weight gain.

When it comes to weight-loss success, "tortoise carbs" are the long-term winners. These are the carbohydrates that slowly raise the blood sugar and enable you to lose weight and prevent or reverse diseases. These low-glycemic tortoise carbs can be broken down into the following groups:

- Vegetables (except potatoes)
- Fruits (except bananas and dried fruits)
- Starches, such as millet bread, brown rice pasta, steel-cut oatmeal, sweet potatoes, new potatoes, brown rice, and wild rice, in small quantities (Minimize these starches; some patients have to eliminate them altogether.)
- Dairy products, such as skim milk; low-fat, low-sugar yogurt; kefir; and low-fat cottage cheese (Minimize dairy products.)
- Legumes, such as beans, peas, lentils, hummus, and peanuts (I recommend 1–4 cups of these starches a day, but start with small servings. You may need Beano, an enzyme that helps you digest beans and minimize gas.)
- Nuts and seeds (raw) (a handful a day)

Even though most of these tortoise carbohydrates are healthy, it's still possible to choose the wrong types of starches and dairy or overeat low-glycemic starches, such as millet bread and brown rice pasta. For this reason, and because there are other ways carbohydrates stall weight-loss efforts, it's important to incorporate the glycemic index and glycemic load principles I discussed in the previous chapter.

> No temptation has overtaken you except such as is common to man; but God is faithful, who will not allow you to be tempted beyond what you are able, but with the temptation will also make the way of escape, that you may be able to bear it.
>
> —1 CORINTHIANS 10:13, NKJV

IS IT A HARE OR A TORTOISE?

The faster your body digests a carbohydrate, the faster it raises your blood sugar—and the higher the glycemic index value of that carb. This is what makes a carb a hare rather than a tortoise. Yet how exactly can you differentiate between the two? Here are a few traits that will help distinguish between a tortoise and a hare.

Fat content. With the exception of seeds, nuts, and dairy, most tortoise carbohydrates are low in fat. Fats are not an inherent evil, as some diets claim. But consuming highly processed, high-fat carbohydrates will sabotage your weight-loss efforts.

Fiber content. Generally a higher fiber content of a food slows down the absorption of sugar, making the carb a tortoise. Beans, peas, and lentils are high in fiber.

Form of starch. Certain starches, such as potatoes, bread, pasta, and white rice, contain amylopectin, which is a complex carbohydrate that the body rapidly absorbs and that usually raises one's blood sugar. However, beans, peas, legumes, and sweet potatoes contain another complex carb called amylose, which is digested more slowly and raises the blood sugar in a slower fashion. Caution is needed with whole-wheat products, as I have discussed. Almost all corn products are considered hare carbohydrates (with a high glycemic index value). Exceptions are corn on the cob and frozen corn, because they are digested more slowly and gradually raise the blood sugar.

Ripeness. The riper the fruit, the faster it is absorbed. For instance, brown, spotted bananas raise blood sugar much faster than regular yellow bananas since they have a higher sugar content.

Cooking. Most brown rice pasta can be either a tortoise carbohydrate or a hare carbohydrate, depending on how you cook it. If you cook it al dente, still leaving it firm, it is typically a tortoise carbohydrate and has a low glycemic index value. Also, thicker pasta noodles generally have a lower glycemic index value than thinner types of pasta (angel hair, thin spaghetti, etc.). Again, I don't recommend any wheat pasta products, even whole grain, since they have a higher glycemic load than many other carbohydrates.

Milling type. A finely ground grain is a hare carbohydrate and has a higher glycemic index value than coarsely ground grain, which has a higher fiber content and thus is a tortoise.

Protein content. The higher the protein content of a food, the more it helps prevent a rapid rise in blood sugar and makes the food more likely to be lower glycemic. Thus it is a tortoise carbohydrate.

A **BIBLE CURE** Health Tip

PGX Fiber

PGX, short for PolyGlycoPlex, is a unique blend of highly viscous fibers that act synergistically to create a much higher level of viscosity than the individual fibers alone. PGX absorbs hundreds of times its weight in water over one to two hours and expands in the digestive tract, creating a thick gelatinous material. It creates a feeling of fullness, stabilizes blood sugar and insulin levels, and stabilizes appetite hormones.

PGX lowers blood sugar after eating by about 20 percent and lowers insulin secretion by about 40 percent. Researchers have found that higher doses of PGX can decrease appetite significantly. PGX works similar to gastric banding and has fewer gastrointestinal side effects than other viscous dietary fibers. However, start slowly, or you may develop gas.

To aid in weight loss, I recommend starting with two or three capsules of PGX fiber with 16 ounces of water before every meal and gradually increasing the dose if needed. This usually prevents you from overeating and enables you to feel satisfied sooner. (See appendix B.)

THE POWER OF PROTEIN

Proteins and amino acids are the building blocks for the body. They are used to repair and maintain tissues such as muscles, connective tissue, our skin, our hair, our bone matrix, and even our nails. If you do not have adequate protein, you will not be able to adequately maintain these tissues I just listed, as well as enzymes, hormones, and your immune system. As a result, you will age faster and eventually develop disease.

> Beloved, I pray that you may prosper in all things and be in health, just as your soul prospers.
>
> —3 JOHN 2, NKJV

But in the same way too many low-glycemic carbs can sabotage your weight-loss goals, so can too much protein have a negative effect on your well-being. Studies have shown that men with diets high in red meat have an increased risk of prostate cancer, and it is typically a more aggressive form of prostate cancer. However, men who eat fish three times a week have approximately half the risk of developing prostate cancer compared to men who rarely eat fish. Also, frying or grilling meat, chicken, or fish so that it is charred or well done is also associated with an increased risk of cancer.

In 2002 the NIH advised that protein should make up 15 to 35 percent of a person's daily consumption of energy or total calories. I believe that anything more than 35 percent of our daily calories as protein is simply too much. I tell my patients to get approximately 15 to 20 percent of their daily calories from protein, but I recommend only 10 percent or less of our calories should come from animal protein. This usually translates into 3 ounces of animal protein once or twice a day for women and 3 to 6 ounces of animal protein once or twice a day for men. Men should limit red meat to only 12 ounces a week. I also strongly believe in consuming some protein with each meal and snack, but realize that we don't need animal protein with each meal. Beans and a small amount of brown rice (the size of a tennis ball) is a complete protein. This helps to create the correct fuel mixture that keeps your appetite controlled, your energy up, and your blood sugar and insulin levels in check—all while your metabolism continues to burn off those extra pounds.

Free-range or organic lean chicken and turkey; organic or omega-3 eggs; wild-caught, low-mercury fish; and organic low-fat dairy are the best choices of animal proteins. These meats are free of hormones and antibiotics that can be harmful to the body. Also, avoid or limit high-fat junk meats such as hot dogs, bologna, salami, pepperoni, and bacon, which are loaded with salt, nitrates, and nitrites. Nitrates and nitrites are associated with an increased risk of certain cancers.

Organic legumes, whole grains, and nuts are the best plant proteins. Vegetarians are able to combine plant proteins with their regular meals to have a high-quality protein. For example, by combining whole grain rice and beans you can form complete proteins. Soy, however, is an exception and is already considered a complete protein.

The potential problem with combining two starches to make a complete protein is that it is easy to slow down or entirely stop your weight loss if your portions are too big. If you can keep this in mind, however, there is no reason you should not enjoy the added benefits and flavors of these proteins. Black bean soup or lentil soup and a small amount of wild rice is a complete protein and very filling—and yes, you will most likely start losing weight if you regularly consume it.

Plant-based protein powder is also a good way to add protein to your meals and snacks. But you should consume soy products with caution. Many scientists now believe that over-consuming soy may do more harm than good. High consumption of isoflavones, which are the estrogen-like plant chemicals contained in soy, may stimulate the production of breast cancer cells. It may also increase the chances of developing serious reproductive, thyroid, and liver problems.[2]

Besides this, most soy products are processed and have a low biological value compared to other proteins—meaning the body doesn't use them very efficiently. This includes two of the most commonly consumed soy products, soy milk and soy protein. These products can interfere with thyroid function and lower the metabolic rate, making it more difficult to lose weight.

I recommend cutting back on soy products if you desire to lose weight. And let me emphasize this: the final word on soy is not yet in. Even the soy skeptics say the bottom line is to opt for natural forms of soy rather than chemically altered or genetically modified (GM). Because it remains a somewhat controversial protein, my advice is to proceed with caution; do not eat or drink soy products every day, but if you must consume soy, do it only a few times a week.

THE TRUTH ABOUT FAT

Too much of any fat—whether good or bad—will make you fat. But overall, fats are critically important for our health. Among their many roles, their main purpose in the body is to provide fuel for cells. Each of the trillions of cells in your body is surrounded by a fatty cell membrane composed primarily of polyunsaturated and saturated fats. The saturated fats provide a rigid support for the cell membrane. The polyunsaturated fats, meanwhile, add flexibility to the cell membranes and allow the transfer of nutrients inside the cells and waste products to be passed outside the cells. These cell membranes need a proper balance of both saturated and polyunsaturated fats.

Likewise, we need a proper balance of fats in our diet to help with the absorption of fat-soluble vitamins, including vitamins A, D, E, and K. We also need fats to produce hormones that regulate inflammation, blood clotting, and muscle contraction. Approximately 60 percent of your brain is composed of fat. You need cholesterol to make brain cells, and most of your cholesterol comes from saturated fats. Fats make up the coverings that surround and protect nerves. They help to satisfy hunger for extended periods. As you can see, fats are not the villains we have made them out to be.

The majority of Americans consume approximately one-third of their total calories from fats. Even though this is a fairly safe amount of fat, Americans continue to gain weight and suffer from an epidemic of being overweight and obese. For this reason, I recommend approximately 25 to 30 percent of your total calorie intake as fats (making sure to choose *good* fats) in order to lose weight.

Bad fats include trans fats and refined omega-6 fats such as most commercial oils, salad dressings, gravies, sauces, and deep-fried foods. Fats that are good in moderation and fats that are bad in excess include saturated fats and unrefined omega-6 fats such as cold-pressed vegetable oils. Good fats include omega-3 fats such as fish oils, flaxseed, salba seed, hemp and chia seed, and oils made from these seeds; monounsaturated fats such as extra-virgin olive oil, avocados, almonds, and other nuts and seeds; and GLA omega-6 fatty acids such as borage oil, evening primrose oil, and black currant seed oil.

I believe no more than 5 to 10 percent of your fat intake should be saturated fats. I strongly recommend that you avoid all trans fats, deep-fried and pan-fried (not stir-fried) foods, and refined omega-6 fats, such as most regular salad dressings, sauces, and gravies. Consuming modest amounts of omega-3 fats, monounsaturated fats, GLA omega-6 fats, and raw seeds and nuts will help decrease insulin resistance, which in turn enables you to lose weight. Our bodies need the proper balance of good healthy oils for all our cells, tissues, and organs to function properly. Fats are not evil; they're essential.

What you eat makes all the difference in the world for your overall well-being! Ask God to give you a new way of looking at nutrition. You'll be surprised at the way your thinking about food begins to change.

A **BIBLE CURE** *Prayer for You*

Lord, I thank You that I am fearfully and wonderfully made. Your Word says we perish for lack of knowledge. Thank You for teaching me about how my body works. Help me to make wise choices so I can lose excess belly fat, be healthy, and function at my best. In Jesus's name, amen.

A **BIBLE CURE** *Prescription*

Take inventory of the foods you typically eat.

- Describe how you will add more good carbohydrates into your diet.

  _____

  _____

- List the foods that you need to eliminate from your diet:

  _____

  _____

- Write a prayer asking God to help you choose foods that will allow your body to function at its best and cause you to lose excess fat:

  _____

  _____

  _____

  _____

Chapter 4

POWER FOR CHANGE
THROUGH DIET AND NUTRITION

WOULD YOU LIKE a supernatural guarantee for success? Here it is: the Bible says to commit your plans to the Lord. "Commit your works to the LORD, and your thoughts will be established" (Prov. 16:3, NKJV). So I want to encourage you to study this plan and then commit it to the Lord for the strength and willpower to follow through.

God is greater than any bondage you may have. And He promises to help you succeed, not with your own power, but by asking for His. He is so faithful. When you ask Him for help, He promises never to fail you or leave you struggling all alone. For the Word of God says, "For He Himself has said, 'I will never leave you nor forsake you'" (Heb. 13:5, NKJV). What a powerful promise!

In this chapter we will look at the eating habits that will lead to healthy, consistent weight loss. But first a word of caution. As I have said before, the number on the scale is not the best measure of weight loss. Make sure you keep the right focus. Instead of focusing on how much you weigh, focus on eating right. When you eliminate sugar, sweets, excessive carbohydrates, bad fats, wheat, and corn from your diet, you will most likely begin to lose weight.

This Bible Cure waist-reducing plan is more than a diet. It is a lifestyle that will help you to look and feel your very best. So, let's get started.

THE MEDITERRANEAN DIET

According to a recent study, "People who eat a Mediterranean-style diet rich in fruits, vegetables, whole grains, olive oil, and fish have at least a 25 percent reduced risk of dying from heart disease and cancer."[1] This is because the Mediterranean diet derives roughly 30 to 40 percent of its calories from healthy fats (coming from foods like olive oil, avocados, nuts, and fish) and about 40 to 50 percent from healthy carbohydrates like fruits, vegetables, beans, peas, lentils, and whole grains. Researchers also surmised that it was not any one component of this diet that makes it preventative, but it's the overall combination of foods, as well as avoiding foods that are potentially harmful, such as excessive calories from omega-6 oils, butter, sweets, and meats.

Combined with daily exercise, this is a powerful diet for living a longer and healthier life. Another study estimated that up to 25 percent of the incidence of colorectal cancer, about 15 percent of the incidence of breast cancer, and about 10 percent of the incidence of prostate cancer could be prevented if we shifted from a common Western diet to a traditional Mediterranean one.[2]

I believe the Mediterranean diet should be the foundation of your daily meal-planning, but you will need to make adjustments. Although breads and pastas are staples of the Mediterranean diet, I highly recommend that you avoid wheat and corn products at least until you have reached your desired waist measurement. You will also need to choose foods that do not create an inflammatory response in your body. But before we discuss what foods to avoid, let's first take a look at the primary foods in the Mediterranean diet. (For a more detailed look at the Mediterranean diet, refer to my books *Dr. Colbert's "I Can Do This" Diet, Eat This and Live!*, and *What Would Jesus Eat?*)

- *Extra-virgin olive oil*—replaces most fats, oils, butter, and margarine. It is used in salads as well as for cooking. Extra-virgin olive oil strengthens the immune system. I recommend 4 tablespoons a day.

- *Bread*—consumed daily and prepared as whole-grain, dark, chewy, crusty loaves. I recommend waiting until you reach your desired weight or waist size to eat bread. At that point, choose whole- and sprouted-grain breads such as Ezekiel 4:9 bread but avoid white processed bread. (I do not recommend wheat or corn until you have achieved your desired waist measurement.)

- *Thick, whole-grain pasta; brown or wild rice; couscous; bulgur; potatoes*—often served with fresh vegetables and herbs, sautéed in olive oil, and occasionally served with small quantities of lean beef. Again, I recommend avoiding pasta and all wheat products to lose weight. Also, limit the other starches to a tennis-ball serving, but no more than one of these starches a meal.

- *Fruit*—preferably raw, two to three pieces daily, but avoid bananas and dried fruit

- *Nuts*—pecans, almonds, cashews, macadamia nuts, hazelnuts, and walnuts; preferably raw, and one handful a day

- *Beans*—including pintos, great northern, navy, black, red, and kidney beans. Hummus, beans, and lentil soups are very popular (prepared with a small amount of extra-virgin olive oil). I recommend at least 1 to 4 cups of beans, peas, lentils, or hummus a day either as a soup or with the entree. (Beano helps prevent gas.)

- *Vegetables*—all types, including dark green variety, especially in salads, or eaten raw or steamed. Eat a large salad with extra-virgin olive oil and vinegar, and choose romaine, spinach, arugala, etc., but do not choose iceberg lettuce. Iceberg lettuce is very low in fiber and nutritional content. Avoid the croutons.

- *Small amounts of low-fat organic cheese and yogurt*— cheese may be grated on soups or entrees. (The reduced-fat cheeses often taste better than the fat-free varieties. The best yogurt is Greek yogurt, fat free, and organic without added fruit, but not frozen.) Also, try grated feta or goat cheese in place of regular cheese.

In addition to eating the foods listed above, the following foods consumed a few times weekly make a good addition to the Mediterranean diet.

- *Fish.* The healthiest fish are cold-water varieties such as cod, wild salmon, sardines, and tongol tuna. These are high in omega-3 fatty acids. Avoid farm-raised fish and high-mercury fish. (See "Bible Cure Health Fact: Mercury Levels in Fish.")

- *Organic or free-range poultry.* Poultry should be eaten two to three times weekly. Eat white breast meat with the skin removed.

- *Organic or omega-3 eggs.* These should be eaten only in small amounts (two to three per week). I recommend eating only one egg yolk with three egg whites and adding veggies to make an omelet once or twice a week and cooked in extra-virgin olive oil.

- *Organic or free-range lean red meat.* Red meat should be eaten only rarely, on an average of once or twice a week. (I suggest consuming less than 12 ounces of red meat a week.) Use only lean cuts with the fat trimmed. Use in small amounts as an additive to spice up soup or pasta. (Note: the severe restriction of red meat in the Mediterranean diet is a radical departure from the American diet, but it is a major contributor to the low rates of cancer, heart disease, and stroke found in these countries.)

A **BIBLE CURE** Health Fact

Dueling Diets

A study published by the *New England Journal of Medicine* found that following a Mediterranean-style diet helped participants reduce their risk of heart attack, stroke, and death from heart disease by 30 percent. In fact, the benefits of the Mediterranean diet on heart health were so clear, the study was stopped early. Conducted in Spain, the study randomly assigned more than 7,000 people who had various risk factors for heart disease including obesity and diabetes to one of three groups. One group followed a low-fat diet, and two groups were put on a Mediterranean diet, eating fish, grains, fruits, and vegetables while avoiding red meats and processed foods. One of the groups assigned to the Mediterranean diet was instructed to eat at least 4 tablespoons of extra-virgin olive oil a day and the other an ounce—or roughly a quarter cup—of walnuts, hazelnuts, and almonds each day. Not only did those on the Mediterranean diet lower their heart disease risk, but they were also able to stay with the diet. The low-fat dieters were not able to stick with the plan and ended up eating a typical modern diet.[3]

A DEADLY BY-PRODUCT OF THE WESTERN DIET: INFLAMMATION

One of the biggest problems with our modern, high-fat, highly processed, high-sugar, high-grain (such as wheat and corn), high-sodium diets is that it has thrown off the balance in our bodies between inflammatory and anti-inflammatory chemicals called *prostaglandins*. Normally inflammation is a good thing that works to repair an injury or fight off infection in the body. It puts the immune system on high alert to attack invading bacteria or viruses to rid our body of these intruders, or in the case of an injury, it rushes white blood cells to the cut, scrape, sprain, or broken bone to remove the damaged cells, splint the injury, or attack infections to facilitate healing.

> Who gives food to all flesh, for His mercy endures forever.
> Oh, give thanks to the God of heaven! For His mercy endures
> forever.
>
> —PSALM 136:25–26, NKJV

This is the good side of inflammation and an extremely important function of the immune system's small agents. When our bodies are in such an emergency, there is a complicated process through which more pro-inflammatory prostaglandins are created than anti-inflammatory ones, and the immune system responds to the sounding of this alarm. When the crisis is over, the balance swings in the anti-inflammatory direction and eventually balances out again.

If you look at this process in a grossly simplified sense, you will see that prostaglandins are produced from the foods we eat in an ongoing cycle, and each of the foods we eat has either a pro-inflammatory tendency or an anti-inflammatory one. Fatty acids are at the center of this. Omega-6 fatty acids are "friendly" to the creation of pro-inflammatory prostaglandins, and omega-3 fatty acids are "friendly" to the creation of anti-inflammatory prostaglandins. A more natural, Mediterranean-type diet will have a balance of pro- and anti-inflammatory-friendly foods; however, our modern high-fat, high-sodium, high-sugar, highly processed Western diet throws that balance off in favor of the production of pro-inflammatory prostaglandins.

Experts tell us that our typical US diet has doubled the amount of omega-6 fatty acids we consume since 1940 as we have shifted more and more away from fruits and vegetables to grain-based foods and the oils produced from them. In fact, we eat about twenty times more omega-6s than we do the anti-inflammatory omega-3s. Most of the animals we obtain food from today are also grain fed, so most of our meats, eggs, and dairy products are higher in omega-6s than they were a century ago. Also, as most of the fish in our stores are now farm raised, they are fed a diet of cereal grains instead of the algae and smaller fish they would live on in the wild, so even our fish are more sources of omega-6s than they used to be. Noting all of this, it is not hard to see why diseases caused by chronic systematic inflammation have grown to be such a problem in the Western world today.

Furthermore, essential fatty acids (EFAs) such as omega-3 and omega-6 cannot be manufactured in the body and must be consumed either through diet or supplements. EFAs help the body repair and create new cells. In addition to reducing inflammation, omega-3 fatty acids can actually create special roadblocks in the body, making it harder for cancer cells to migrate from a primary tumor to start new colonies. Cancers that remain localized in one place are much easier to treat than those that metastasize (spread throughout the body).[4]

Because of the high omega-6 content of our diets, our bodies find more material for pro- than anti-inflammatory prostaglandins. Over time the natural, ongoing creation of prostaglandins will tip the balance toward systematic inflammation as more pro-inflammatory prostaglandins are produced than anti-inflammatory ones. Despite the absence of an actual emergency, this imbalance still sets off alarms calling for chronic or long-term inflammation, and the immune system will respond accordingly. However, with no actual threat present, the immune system will start attacking things it normally wouldn't. This immune hypersensitivity can lead to a glut of problems ranging from simple allergies and weight gain to cancer, Alzheimer's disease, cardiovascular disease, diabetes, arthritis, asthma, prostate problems, and autoimmune diseases.

Many of these happen because as the immune system stays on high alert longer than it should, its agents begin to fatigue and make bad decisions, possibly leading to autoimmune disease or not destroying mutated cells, leading to cancer formation with more frequency. This can easily give way to cancer getting a foothold it won't easily relinquish.

> And my God shall supply all your need according to His riches in glory by Christ Jesus.
> —PHILIPPIANS 4:19, NKJV

Omega-3 fatty acids are clearly incredibly beneficial. Here are some omega-3 foods to include in your diet: flaxseeds and flaxseed oil, chia seeds, salba seeds, hemp seeds, fish (wild salmon, sardines, tongol tuna, herring, and cod), and fish oil. (See Bible Cure Health Fact: Mercury Levels in Fish.) Obviously, it's important to know which fats to eat and which ones to avoid when it comes to preventing those harmful prostaglandins I mentioned above.

So, while using an understanding of the Mediterranean diet as a foundation, within that framework you should also look at how pro-inflammatory or anti-inflammatory the foods you eat are as well. If you are having problems with allergies, joint pains, muscle aches, or the like, by eating more anti-inflammatory foods than pro-inflammatory ones, you can tip your balance back in the right direction.

One way to check your degree of inflammation is to have a C-reactive protein blood test. C-reactive protein is a promoter of inflammation and also a blood marker of systemic inflammation. Once you reach forty years of age, annual CRP testing is a great idea for checking the anti-inflammatory effectiveness of your diet. Men should aim for a CRP less than 1.0, while women should aim for a CRP less than 1.5.

A **BIBLE CURE** Health Fact

Mercury Levels in Fish

Although fish is generally a good protein choice, some fish contain high levels of mercury. The following list will help you determine which fish to eat more liberally and which to avoid.[5]

Fish with least amounts of mercury (enjoy these fish)

- Anchovies
- Catfish
- Crab
- Flounder
- Haddock (Atlantic)
- Herring
- Salmon (fresh or canned)
- Sardines
- Shrimp
- Sole
- Tilapia
- Trout (freshwater)
- Whitefish

Fish with moderate amounts of mercury (eat six servings or less per month)

- Bass (striped or black)
- Halibut (Atlantic or Pacific)
- Lobster
- Mahi-Mahi
- Monkfish
- Snapper
- Tuna (canned, chunk light)

Fish high in mercury (eat three servings or less per month)

- Bluefish
- Grouper
- Mackerel (Spanish and Gulf)
- Sea bass (Chilean)
- Tuna (canned albacore)
- Tuna (yellowfin)

Fish highest in mercury (avoid)

- Mackerel (king)
- Marlin
- Orange roughy
- Shark
- Swordfish
- Tilefish
- Tuna (bigeye and ahi)

THE ANTI-INFLAMMATORY DIET: TAKING THE MEDITERRANEAN DIET TO THE NEXT LEVEL

Using the Mediterranean diet as the foundation for your day-in, day-out meal planning, you can then balance your pro-inflammatory and anti-inflammatory foods as your body (and CRP tests if you have taken them) indicates that you should. This will, of course, initially probably mean adding more anti-inflammatory foods and avoiding the pro-inflammatory ones for a time.

I have organized the following two lists of foods for you to consider adding or subtracting from your diet as your level of systematic inflammation demands.

TOP ANTI-INFLAMMATORY FOODS (ALWAYS CHOOSE ORGANIC WHEN POSSIBLE)	
Fruit	Raspberries, acerola (West Indian) cherries, guava, strawberries, cantaloupe, lemons/limes, rhubarb, kumquat, pink grapefruit, mulberries, blueberries, blackberries
Vegetables	Chili peppers, onions (including scallions and leeks), spinach, greens (including kale, collards, and turnip and mustard greens), sweet potatoes, carrots, garlic
Legumes	Lentils, green beans, peas
Egg products	Liquid eggs, egg whites (may use one organic or free-range egg yolk with three egg whites)
Dairy (use with caution)	Cottage cheese (low fat and nonfat), nonfat cream cheese, plain low-fat Greek yogurt or vanilla Greek yogurt (add fresh fruit if desired) (Limit dairy to 4–6 oz. every three to four days)
Fish	Herring, haddock, wild salmon (not farmed; Alaskan preferred), rainbow trout, sardines, anchovies (See Bible Cure Health Fact: Mercury Levels in Fish.)
Poultry	Goose, duck, free-range organic chicken and turkey (white meat preferred, skins removed) (3–6 oz. once or twice a day)
Meat	Eye of round (beef), flank steak, sirloin tip, skirt steak, pork tenderloin (free range preferred, extra lean or lean) (Limit to 3–6 oz. two times a week, 12 oz. max.)
Cereal	Steel-cut oatmeal, oat bran
Fats/oils	Safflower oil (high oleic), hazelnut oil, extra-virgin olive oil, avocado oil, almond oil, apricot kernel oil
Nuts/seeds	Brazil nuts, macadamia nuts, hazelnuts, pecans, almonds, hickory nuts, cashews (best raw)
Herbs/spices	Garlic, onion, cayenne, ginger, turmeric, chili peppers, chili powder, curry powder, rosemary, boswellia
Sweeteners	Stevia, tagatose, coconut palm sugar
Beverages	Black, white, or green tea, club soda/seltzer, herbal tea, spring water
Starches	Sweet potatoes, new potatoes, millet bread, brown and wild rice, brown rice pasta, and legumes (see above for approved legumes)

INFLAMMATORY FOODS TO LIMIT OR AVOID	
Fruit	Mango, banana, dried apricots, dried apples, dried dates, canned fruits, raisins
Vegetables	White potatoes, french fries, potato chips
Legumes	Baked beans, fava beans (boiled), canned beans
Egg products	Duck eggs, goose eggs, hard-boiled eggs, egg yolks
Cheeses	Brick cheese, cheddar cheese, Colby cheese, cream cheese (normal and reduced fat)
Dairy	Fruited yogurt, ice cream, butter
Fish	Farm-raised fish and fish high in mercury (See Bible Cure Health Fact: Mercury Levels in Fish.)
Poultry	Turkey (dark meat), Cornish game hen, chicken giblets, chicken liver
Meat	Bacon, veal loin, veal kidney, beef lung, beef kidney, beef heart, beef brain, pork chitterlings, lamb rib chops, dark turkey meat with skin, turkey wing with skin, all processed meats
Breads	Hot dog/hamburger buns, English muffins, Kaiser rolls, bagels, french bread, Vienna bread, blueberry muffins, oat bran muffins
Cereal	Grape-Nuts, Crispix, Corn Chex, Just Right, Rice Chex, corn flakes, Rise Krispies, Raisin Bran, shredded wheat
Pasta/grain	White rice, lasagna noodles, macaroni elbows, regular pasta, all corn products except corn on the cob or frozen corn (non-GMO)
Fats/oils	Margarine, wheat germ oil, sunflower oil, poppy seed oil, grape seed oil, safflower oil, cottonseed oil, palm kernel oil, corn oil
Sweeteners	Honey, brown sugar, white sugar, corn syrup, powdered sugar
Crackers/ chips/ cookies	Corn chips, pretzels, graham crackers, saltines, vanilla wafers
Desserts	Sweetened condensed milk, angel food cake, chocolate and vanilla cake with frosting, chocolate chips, heavy whipping cream, ice cream, fruit leather snacks (Most all desserts are made with sugar.)
Candy	Hershey Kisses, jelly beans, Twix, Almond Joy, milk chocolate bars, Snickers
Beverages	Milk, Gatorade, pineapple juice, orange juice, cranberry juice, lemonade, sodas, sugar-laden soft drinks

These are not complete lists by any means—just some of the more likely "suspects" to watch out for and some of the more helpful helpers to work into your diet. As you read these now, some of them will jump out at you as things you like and need, but you don't have as much of them in your diet as you probably should. Others are the foods that it is time to change your habits about and say good-bye to. The thing to remember is that you have a choice about what you put in your mouth, and now that you have a little more knowledge about these foods, you can begin making healthier diet choices concerning them.

If you have no health problems or obesity, avoiding the inflammatory foods on the previous pages is a good general guideline, and simply follow the Mediterranean diet I outlined earlier. Because your health is good, you have a little more freedom than someone who is struggling with his or her health or weight. You may eat some of the inflammatory foods listed, but I highly recommend you use moderation when consuming them.

> I will instruct you and teach you in the way you should go; I will guide you with My eye.
>
> —PSALM 32:8, NKJV

If you have health problems or obesity, then in addition to understanding the anti-inflammatory and inflammatory food lists on the previous pages, I advise you to adhere to the following anti-inflammatory diet exactly as directed below and avoid all inflammatory foods. Once your health conditions clear up or you are able to maintain a healthy weight, you can ease up on the following guidelines. If you reintroduce wheat into your diet, choose whole-grain breads and sprouted breads such as Ezekiel 4:9 bread, and avoid white processed bread. But again use moderation whenever eating inflammatory foods.

DR. COLBERT'S ANTI-INFLAMMATORY DIET (ALWAYS CHOOSE ORGANIC WHEN POSSIBLE)	
Vegetables	• Steam, stir fry, or cook under low heat. • Best cooked with extra-virgin olive oil, macadamia nut oil, or coconut oil • Vegetable soups should be non-cream-based, low sodium (homemade is best); you may add some organic meat. • Juice your own vegetable juice; avoid store-bought juices, which are usually high in sodium.
Animal proteins (meat)	• 3 oz. once or twice a day for women; 3 to 6 oz. once or twice a day for men • Wild salmon, sardines, anchovies, tongol tuna, turkey (skin removed), free-range chicken (skin removed), eggs (omega-3 eggs as well) • When grilling, slice meat into thin slices; marinate in red wine, pomegranate juice, cherry juice, or curry sauce. Remove all char from meat. • Be cautious with egg yolks, keeping to a maximum of once or twice a week. You can combine one yolk with two to three egg whites. • Limit consumption of lean beef and red meat to one to two 3 to 6 oz. servings a week.
Fruits	• Berries, Granny Smith apples, lemon, or lime. If diabetic, choose only berries.
Nuts and seeds	• All raw nuts and seeds are acceptable, but just a handful once or twice a day.
Salads	• Use 1-calorie-per-spray salad spritzers; or create your own vinaigrette spritzer using a one to two ratio of extra-virgin olive oil to balsamic, apple cider, or red wine vinegar. So you would mix 1 to 2 Tbsp. extra-virgin olive oil with 2 to 4 Tbsp. vinegar. Once you attain a healthy weight and waistline, increase your olive oil to 4 Tbsp. a day in your salad dressing.
Dairy	• Low-fat dairy without sugar such as Greek yogurt and low-fat cottage cheese

DR. COLBERT'S ANTI-INFLAMMATORY DIET (ALWAYS CHOOSE ORGANIC WHEN POSSIBLE)	
Starches	• Sweet potatoes, new potatoes, brown/wild rice, millet bread, brown rice pasta • Two to four cups daily of beans, peas, legumes, lentils, or hummus • Use moderation when choosing starches, at most only one serving per meal, and make them the size of a tennis ball, not a basketball. • If diabetic, I recommend that you avoid starches.
Beverages	• Alkaline water or sparkling water; may add lemon or lime • Green, black, or white tea; may add lemon or lime • Coffee • Low-fat coconut milk or almond milk in place of cow's milk • No sugar; use stevia or other sugar substitutes such as Just Like Sugar, Sweet Balance, xylitol, chicory, or tagatose or coconut palm sugar in moderation. • No cream; use low-fat coconut milk.
Avoid	• Avoid all gluten (wheat, barley, rye, spelt); this includes all products made with these grains, including bread, pasta, crackers, bagels, pretzels, most cereals, etc. Go to www.celiacsociety.com for gluten-free foods. Also avoid corn products except for corn on the cob. Choose non-GMO.
Avoid	• Inflammatory animal proteins such as shellfish, pork, lamb, veal, and organ meats • Sugar • Fried foods • Processed foods • High-glycemic foods such as white rice, instant potatoes, etc.

Be sure to rotate your vegetables and meats every four days if you have food sensitivities. Do not eat the same food every day.

A **BIBLE CURE** *Health Fact*

Choose Olive Oil Wisely

Do not buy extra-virgin olive oil packaged in a large plastic bottle. Olive oil is perishable, or it turns rancid. You should buy small amounts, packaged in dark glass bottles, and store it in a dark pantry at a cool temperature. Check expiration dates, and throw it away if it smells or tastes rancid.

A WORD ABOUT PORTION SIZES

Any plan to lose weight will require you to limit your portions, but that doesn't mean you have to feel deprived. Barbara Rolls, PhD, introduced the concept of "volumetrics" as an answer to dieters who were sick of always feeling hunger. Her premise is simple: rather than eating tiny amounts of calorie-dense foods, eat lots of low-calorie foods that are naturally rich in water and fiber. Instead of bothering with counting calories or grams of fat, protein, or carbs, Rolls argues that dieters can eat more than they normally do and still lose weight—as long as they eat the right type of foods (ones that aren't calorie-dense).

Though I differ on many of her points, I believe Rolls is onto something by understanding that you can eat large portions of foods with little to no calories. Vegetables are a perfect example of this, which is why in this Bible Cure program you are essentially able to eat as many vegetables as you want with meals (minus the butter, of course). In fact, there are a few simple volumetric tips you can use at every meal.

- Before every meal drink a tall glass of water with two or three capsules of PGX fiber. This usually prevents you from overeating.

- Enjoy a bowl of vegetable soup, minestrone soup, black bean soup, lentil soup, or any other broth-based, low-sodium, non-cream-based vegetable soup. A study done at Penn State concluded that eating a bowl of soup with an entree actually reduced the total

consumed calories by 20 percent.[6] A cup of bean, pea,
or lentil soup before your meal is very filling and will
help you lose weight, but eat no more than four cups
of beans, peas, and lentils per day.

- Precede your entree with a salad (any size). Make sure
  you use a salad spritzer with 1 calorie per spray. If
  you decide to eat your salad with extra-virgin olive
  oil and vinegar, be sure to limit your olive oil to 1 to
  2 tablespoons and two or three times as much vinegar.
  You will use less if you use a salad spritzer. Avoid the
  croutons.

- Whether eating a salad or your entree, always
  remember to chew every bite twenty to thirty times;
  this not only helps your body digest and absorb the
  food's nutrients, but it also causes you to eat slower
  and fill up faster.

By prefilling your stomach with low-calorie foods, you are less
likely to eat excess amounts of starches, meats, fats, and desserts.

SNACKING RIGHT

Ideally, you should eat every three to three and a half hours to avoid
hunger. Many people do not understand that a good snack can turn
off your appetite and can stop the triggers from setting it off in the
first place. And though it seems counterintuitive to some, snacking
can help you burn more calories in the process. Researchers have
determined that snacking on the right amount of healthy foods, in
addition to eating three meals a day, boosts the metabolic rate more
than if you only eat three meals each day.[7]

The best type of snack food is a mini-meal consisting of healthy protein; a high-fiber, low-glycemic carbohydrate or starch; and some good
fat. When mixed together, this food fuel or fuel mixture is digested
slowly, causing glucose to trickle into your bloodstream, which controls your hunger for hours. Portion control is a key to wise snacking.
Select half a serving of either a low-glycemic starch or one serving size
of fruit. Then add 1 to 2 ounces of a protein and a third of a serving
size of healthy fat. Typically this mini-meal should amount to just

100 to 150 calories for women and 150 to 250 calories for men. Here are a few examples of well-rounded snacks.

Morning or afternoon snack

- 2 tablespoons of guacamole or avocado with raw carrots or celery
- 2 tablespoons of hummus with raw carrots or celery (4 inches in length)
- 10–15 baked lentil chips and 2 tablespoons of hummus, guacamole, or avocado (You can purchase the baked lentil chips at www.mediterranean snackfoods.com.)
- 1 to 2 wedges of Laughing Cow Light cheese, 1 ounce of smoked salmon or tongol tuna (meat optional)
- Half a cup of nonfat cottage cheese, a piece of low-glycemic fruit (berries or Granny Smith apple), and 5 to 10 nuts
- A small salad with 1 to 2 ounces of sliced turkey (optional) and 2 tablespoons of avocado; in a salad spritzer combine 1 tablespoon extra-virgin olive oil and 2 to 3 tablespoons vinegar
- A bowl of broth-based vegetable, lentil, or bean soup with 1 to 2 ounces of boiled chicken
- A protein smoothie made from plant protein powder (1–2 scoops) mixed with 2 to 4 ounces of frozen berries and 8 ounces of low-fat coconut or almond milk, or coconut kefir (option: dilute the coconut milk, almond milk, or kefir by reducing it to 4 ounces and combining with 4 ounces of filtered water or spring water)

Evening snacks

- Protein drink
- Lettuce wraps

- Salad with or without lean meat (may use a salad
  spritzer or one part extra-virgin olive oil mixed with
  two to three parts vinegar)

- Vegetable or bean or lentil soup with or without lean
  meat

Be sure to take two or three PGX fiber capsules with a 16-ounce glass of water with your snack. And remember you can add as many non-starchy vegetables as you want. To top it off, I recommend a cup of green or black tea, using natural stevia as a sweetener.

> "Not by might nor by power, but by My Spirit," says the Lord
> of hosts.
>
> —Zechariah 4:6, NKJV

Keep plenty of healthy snack items at home, at work, and on the road. Always be prepared. And don't forget: it is important to get snacks that you truly enjoy. Otherwise you won't bother.

A **Bible Cure** Health Fact

Timely Eating

Research has shown that people who successfully lose weight and keep it off eat breakfast every day. Other studies have gone a step further, proving that people who skip breakfast are prone to eating more food and snacks during the day.[8]

Unfortunately, most Americans have their meals backward. We skimp on breakfast, eat a medium-size lunch, and then pig out come dinnertime. We should actually be doing the opposite. As the saying goes, we should eat breakfast like a king (within thirty minutes of waking up), lunch like a prince, and dinner like a pauper.

Eat every three to three and a half hours to avoid hunger. Eating at the right times will leave you energized, mentally sharper, and more emotionally stable. Even your job performance will go up as a result.

ACCELERATING YOUR WEIGHT LOSS

For those who need to quickly lose weight to ward off or reverse obesity-related illness such as diabetes, I developed the Rapid Waist Reduction Diet. This plan is based on protocol Dr. A. T. W. Simeons developed more than sixty years ago. He found that when his 500-calorie-a-day, very low-fat and very low-carbohydrate diet was combined with small daily doses of the pregnancy hormone hCG (human chorionic gonadotropin), it caused the body to release abnormal collections of fat in the problem areas of the hips, thighs, buttocks, waist, and belly.

In Dr. Simeons's day patients were hospitalized for in-patient treatment for the entire six-week duration of the program. According to Dr. Simeons, 60 to 70 percent of the patients kept the weight off long-term.

Many consider Dr. Simeons's protocol the best-kept medical secret as well as the most effective weight-loss program of all time. In 2007 consumer advocate Kevin Trudeau made Dr. Simeons's protocol known to the world in his book *The Weight Loss Cure "They" Don't Want You to Know About.* I started recommending the Simeons Protocol and monitoring patients back in 2008. At that time I used hCG injections. However, now I recommend either the sublingual hCG tab that is compounded by a compounding pharmacy or homeopathic hCG drops.*

The Food and Drug Administration (FDA) requires us to inform patients of the following statement: "hCG has not been demonstrated to be an effective adjunctive therapy in the treatment of obesity. There is no substantial evidence that it increases weight loss beyond that resulting from calorie restriction, that it causes a more attractive or 'normal' distribution of fat or that it decreases the hunger and discomfort associated with calorie restricted diets."

---

* As of the printing of this book, the FDA does not allow over-the-counter (OTC) hCG drops to be labeled as homeopathic and make claims about weight loss. It is extremely difficult to get homeopathic hCG drops due to the new FDA regulations The drops I recommend have been modified to comply with the FDA. The prescription sublingual hCG tabs I recommend also comply with the FDA restrictions as they are prescribed and not OTC and this new regulation does not pertain to the prescription sublingual hCG drops.

I have modified the 500 calories in the Simeons Protocol to approximately 1,000 calories in my Rapid Waist Reduction Diet, but I've kept Simeons's ratio of proteins, fats, and carbohydrates the same. I also added more soluble fiber and supplements to boost serotonin levels and help with satiety, blood sugar control, and improved bowel movements. Results vary from person to person, but a number of my patients have been able to come off all their medications after following the Rapid Waist Reduction Diet and losing belly fat.

This program is not for everyone. Women who are breastfeeding, pregnant, or planning to become pregnant; those who recently had surgery or cancer; and individuals who have been diagnosed with heart failure, type 1 diabetes, chronic renal failure, severe anemia, mental illness, or any seizure disorders should not participate in this diet plan. Those taking diuretics, anti-inflammatory medications, Coumadin, insulin, or birth control may also be unable to participate.

I believe that anyone should talk with their health care provider before beginning a strict diet or exercise program, but those who are prediabetic or diabetic *must* involve their physicians to ensure the steps they take to incorporate the principles in the Rapid Waist Reduction Diet will work with their particular health needs. If you think this diet is right for you, I encourage you to get my book *The Rapid Waist Reduction Diet*, in which I outline this plan in its entirety.

DON'T GIVE UP

You may think it's impossible for you to lose weight, but with God's help you will get to your goal weight and stay there. Instead of focusing on your weight, focus on the lifestyle and dietary changes you need to make. And don't allow yourself to get stuck thinking you will never succeed at weight loss. Start every day with prayer to God for success. Speak aloud the Bible verses that are scattered throughout this book. In addition, plan your menu each day. With a little patience, you'll be well on your way to becoming the slimmer, healthy person God intended you to be!

A **BIBLE CURE** Prayer for You

Lord, give me the will and determination to eat right and lose weight. Break the bondage of obesity in my life that keeps me from enjoying an abundant life in Christ. Let me be filled with Your strength and power to follow a healthy lifestyle and eat the right foods so that I may serve and love You with my whole heart. Amen.

 ## A **BIBLE CURE** Prescription

Keep a Daily Food Diary

Researchers say that self-monitoring devices, such as a pedometer, heart rate monitor, or even a simple exercise journal, can account for a 25 percent increase in successfully controlling your weight.[9] I encourage you to keep a food journal to monitor your waist measurement, your body fat percentage, what you eat, and to log how often you exercise. I have included a sample food diary. Make copies as needed.

To boost your efforts, find a photograph of yourself at or near a healthy or desired weight and put it in your food journal. As you carry your food journal (see below for a sample) with you throughout the day and look at the picture, visualize yourself becoming that ideal weight again. Confession helps too; each day confess that, by faith, you weigh your desired weight.

Date/Weight and Waist Size	Breakfast	Lunch	Dinner

Chapter 5

TIPS FOR EATING OUT

THE NATIONAL RESTAURANT Association estimates Americans spend 49 percent of their food budget at restaurants.[1] With America's fast-paced lifestyle, many parents feel they do not have time to prepare family meals, leading to an unhealthy reliance on fast-food restaurants. Meanwhile singles or couples without children at home have discovered that eating out regularly is easier and may be more economical. I don't recommend that you eat out all the time, but all of us will eat out from time to time—it is part of modern life.

The good news is that you can eat out and still enjoy a balanced, healthy meal. Most restaurants serve unhealthy food, so you can't eat just anything. In addition, portion sizes are often distorted. If you hope to control your weight, there are basic principles you must understand when deciding what dishes to order at restaurants.

- Choose sparkling water or unsweetened tea with a wedge of lemon or lime.

- Take two to four PGX fiber capsules with 16 ounces of unsweetened tea or water to help prevent overeating.

- Avoid the bread. If possible, ask that it not even be placed on the table.

- Choose an appetizer with vegetables and meats such as a shrimp cocktail. Avoid any that are deep-fried, high in starch and fats (i.e., quesadillas or corn bread), or bread based.

- Order your salad with the dressing on the side and with no croutons, cheese, or fattening side items. It's best to bring your own salad dressing spritzer or use olive oil and vinegar.

- Have a bowl of broth-based vegetable, bean, or lentil soup to fill yourself up before starting your entrée.

- Choose entrées with meat, fish, or poultry that is baked, broiled, grilled, or stir-fried in a minimum amount of oil. Avoid anything deep fried or pan-fried. Meat portion sizes should be 3 ounces for women and 3 to 6 ounces for men. If the portion is larger, ask the server to put half in a to-go box.

- Limit sauces and gravies. If you must have them, ask that they be put on the side.

- Ask that vegetables be steamed without butter or oils (unless you prefer them raw).

- Choose sweet potato over white potato when possible. Because these are high-glycemic foods, keep portion to the size of a tennis ball.

- If you choose a dessert, share it and only take a few bites. Savor those bites.

One of the easiest ways to avoid sabotaging your weight-loss goals is planning. This will help you avoid unhealthy foods and overeating. Never go out to eat when you feel ravenous. I guarantee that you will eat too much of the wrong foods. Have a healthy snack such as a large Granny Smith apple or a pear before leaving the house. This will pre-fill your stomach and help prevent overeating.

In addition, plan what and where you will eat before leaving home. I also suggest patients plan an early dinner, usually between five and six o'clock, so they will finish early enough to burn off some calories before going to bed. You may also want to consider sharing an entrée with your spouse. Also, be sure to slow down while eating, and chew every bite thoroughly, putting your fork down between bites. All these "little" things go a long way in controlling hunger and weight.

SPECIALITY RESTAURANTS

Here are some additional tips to help you make wise choices when eating out at specialty food restaurants.

> But the fruit of the Spirit is love, joy, peace, longsuffering, kindness, goodness, faithfulness, gentleness, self-control.
> —GALATIANS 5:22–23, NKJV

Fast-food restaurants

Choose a grilled chicken sandwich or a small hamburger. Throw away the top and bottom bun, and squeeze your burger between two napkins to remove excess grease. Cut the hamburger in half and then place both halves of the meat between two lettuce leafs. Avoid mayonnaise and ketchup; choose mustard, tomato, onions, and pickle. You can also order a small salad and ask for fat-free dressing (or use just a small portion of a regular packet). For a drink, order unsweetened iced tea or a bottle of water. Instead of french fries, order a baked potato when available, using only one pat of butter or 2 teaspoons of sour cream.

If you eat at a sub shop, choose turkey, lean roast beef, and chicken instead of bologna, pastrami, salami, corned beef, or other fatty selections. Choose a 6-inch sub, eating it with the smaller bottom of the bun and not the top portion. Use plenty of vegetables, and top with vinegar; avoid or go easy on the oil. It's best to further cut calories by ordering it in a lettuce or pita wrap.

At fast-food chicken restaurants, choose rotisserie or baked chicken instead of fried. Peel off the skin and pat the chicken dry with a napkin. Drain the liquid from the coleslaw, and do not eat the biscuit or potatoes.

Before diving into a slice of pizza, eat a large salad. Then have only one slice of pizza, sticking to thin or flatbread crust. Choose chunky tomatoes and other veggies as toppings. Avoid pepperoni and other highly processed meat toppings, and ask for half the cheese (the same way many ask for double cheese). Finally, use a napkin to remove excess oils from the cheese.

Italian restaurants

Start with a soup—minestrone, pasta fagioli, or broth-based tomato—and a large salad. Limit bread and olive oil, which has 120 calories per tablespoon. Good entrée options include grilled chicken, fish, shellfish, veal, and steak. Avoid fried or Parmesan dishes, such as chicken or veal Parmesan. Ask for your vegetables to be steamed, and avoid the pasta or have it cooked al dente, which causes it to have a lower glycemic index value. Don't overdo it on the pasta; the amount should be about the size of a tennis ball. Avoid fat-filled creamy sauces, cheese, and pesto sauce.

Mexican restaurants

Avoid the deep-fried tortilla chips, and choose tortilla soup without the chips or black bean soup as appetizers. Be wary of entrées smothered in melted cheese, which automatically increases the fat count. Choose fajitas with chicken, beef, or shrimp. Avoid the tortilla, and make your fajita with lettuce wraps. Add such ingredients as salsa, onions, lettuce, beans, and guacamole. Avoid cheese and sour cream if possible, since restaurants rarely serve nonfat varieties. As for beans, choose red or black but not refried, since they are high in fat. Avoid the rice. If a salad is available, enjoy a large one before your entrée.

Asian restaurants

These are usually good choices, provided your meat or seafood is baked, steamed, poached, or stir-fried. Steaming is usually the healthiest method. Instead of fried rice or fried noodles, choose brown rice. If permitted, substitute a serving of rice with vegetables. If that is not possible, don't eat more than a tennis-ball-sized serving of rice. Avoid sweet and sour, batter-fried, or twice-cooked food (which is high in fat and calories) and oily sauces (i.e., duck). For an appetizer you can choose wonton or egg drop soup instead of deep-fried egg rolls. Sushi is fine; some restaurants prepare it with brown rice.

Look for restaurants that do not use MSG or that will not use it on your dish. MSG has numerous potential reactions. The most common is stimulating your appetite, causing you to become hungry again in a couple hours. More importantly, MSG can lead to severe headaches, heart palpitations, and shortness of breath. (For more information on MSG, refer to my book *The Seven Pillars of Health*.)

Indian restaurants

Many Indian foods contain large portions of ghee (clarified butter) or oil, so it's best to find a restaurant willing to limit the amount they use on your dish. Tandoori-cooked (roasted) or grilled fish, chicken, beef, and shrimp are good choices. Avoid deep-fried foods and sauces, such as marsala sauce and curry sauce, which are high in fat. If you must have them, get them in a small side dish. Also, it's best to avoid the breads—a major element of Indian food. If you have any, however, choose bread that is baked (*nan*) instead of the fried *chapatis* bread.

Family-style restaurants

Foods at these restaurants are typically high in fats; the main courses are often fried. The vegetables are usually loaded with gravy, butter, or oil. Good choices include baked or grilled chicken, turkey, or beef with steamed vegetables. Vegetable or bean or lentil soup and a salad (dressing on the side) also make good choices. Avoid the large dinner rolls, butter, and fried side dishes. Choose beans, such as lima, pinto, or string beans. If you must have gravy, get it on the side and eat it sparingly. Though raised on Southern cooking, I have learned I can enjoy the foods without all the gravies and fried options.

> The LORD is my strength and my shield; my heart trusted in Him, and I am helped; therefore my heart greatly rejoices, and with my song I will praise Him.
>
> —PSALM 28:7, NKJV

A FINAL WORD

Eating healthily is not a diet but a lifestyle. So follow this lifestyle every day. There will be times that you will slip, especially on holidays, birthdays, anniversaries, weddings, and other special occasions. However, never give up. Simply get back on the program, and you will again start burning fat and building muscle.

If you reach a plateau or if you are unable to lose more weight, simply avoid high-glycemic carbohydrates, which include breads, pasta, potatoes, corn, rice, pretzels, bagels, crackers, cereals, popcorn, beans, bananas, and dried fruit. Choose low-glycemic vegetables and fruits. If after a month or two of doing this you are still unable to lose sufficient weight, you should choose low-glycemic vegetables and salads and avoid fruits for approximately a month until you break through the plateau. Then reintroduce low-glycemic fruits.

I am praying for God to give you the determination and will power to follow through on this eating strategy. Not only will you lose weight, but also you will keep it off. In doing so, you will take care of your body, God's temple, and live a full and abundant life to His glory. Eat right and live in divine health!

A **BIBLE CURE** Prayer for You

Lord, You are my strength. I trust You to help me make healthy choices to reach and maintain a healthy weight even when I am away from home or celebrating with friends and family. I can cry out to You when I am tempted, and You will be there to help me. You never give me more than I can bear. I declare that I will walk in discipline and stay focused on maintaining a healthy lifestyle. In Jesus's name, amen.

A **BIBLE CURE** Prescription

Check the healthy choices you are willing to make when you are eating out:

❑ Plan ahead.

❑ Eat a snack beforehand and/or take PGX fiber supplements.

❑ Take half of my entrée to go.

❑ Avoid dessert.

❑ Other: _____

Write a prayer asking God for help in making wise choices when eating out:

_____

_____

_____

_____

Chapter 6

POWER FOR CHANGE THROUGH ACTIVITY

G OD HAS MADE you the master of your body—it is not the master of you! Too many of us let our bodies tell us what to do. However, God created this incredible body to be your servant. The apostle Paul revealed his understanding of this truth when he said, "I discipline my body and bring it into subjection, lest, when I have preached to others, I myself should become disqualified" (1 Cor. 9:27, NKJV).

God has given you the power of mastery over your body. If you've let it get out of shape, it's time to assert your power!

> And let us not grow weary while doing good, for in due season we shall reap if we do not lose heart.
> —GALATIANS 6:9, NKJV

Proper nutrition alone cannot reduce your weight sufficiently or adequately maintain your proper weight. However, proper nutrition combined with exercise will help you reach your goal of walking in divine health and living a long, wholesome life.

GET MOVING

There is no better way to complement a weight-loss dietary and supplement program than physical activity. It helps raise the metabolic rate during and after the activity. It enables you to develop more muscle, which raises the metabolic rate all day—even while you sleep. It decreases body fat and improves your ability to cope with stress by lowering the stress hormone cortisol.

Such activity also raises serotonin levels, which helps reduce cravings for sweets and carbohydrates. It assists in burning off dangerous belly fat and improves your body's ability to handle sugar. Finally, regular physical activity can even help control your appetite by boosting serotonin levels, lowering cortisol, and decreasing insulin levels (which can also decrease your chances for insulin resistance). Simply put, regular activity is extremely important if you want to lose weight and keep it off.

It's important to see your personal physician before starting a rigorous exercise program. Even if you have health considerations, you may be surprised to learn there are ways for you to become more active. Cycling, swimming, dancing, hiking, and sports such as basketball, volleyball, soccer, and tennis are all considered aerobic. Washing the car by hand, working in your yard, and mowing the grass qualify too. An aerobic exercise is simply something that uses large muscle groups of the body and raises the heart rate to a range that will burn fat for fuel. This is why aerobic exercise is one of the best ways to lose body fat.

A **BIBLE CURE** Health Tip

The Perks of Regular Activity

In case you needed a reminder, here are some of the many benefits that regular activity promotes:

- It decreases the risk of heart disease, stroke, and the development of hypertension.
- It helps prevent type 2 diabetes.
- It helps protect you from developing certain types of cancer.
- It helps prevent osteoporosis and aids in maintaining healthy bones.
- It helps prevent arthritis and aids in maintaining healthy joints.
- It slows down the overall aging process.
- It improves your mood and reduces the symptoms of anxiety and depression.
- It increases energy and mental alertness.
- It improves digestion.

- It gives you more restful sleep.

- It helps prevent colds and flu.

- It alleviates pain.

- It promotes weight loss and decreases appetite.

Try brisk walking. Brisk walking is the simplest and most convenient way to exercise aerobically. Walk briskly enough so that you can't sing, yet slow enough so that you can talk. This is a simple way to ensure you are entering your target heart rate zone. Diabetic patients with foot ulcers or numbness in the feet may want to avoid walking and should try cycling, an elliptical machine, or pool activities while inspecting the feet before and after activity.

Aerobic exercise will make you feel better immediately by putting more oxygen into your body. It also tones the heart and blood vessels, increases circulation, boosts the metabolic rate, improves digestion and elimination, controls insulin production, stimulates the production of neurotransmitters in the brain, improves the appetite and stimulates the lymphatic system, which aids in the removal of toxic material from the body.

Whatever activity you choose, the important thing is that you get moving regularly. Don't give yourself an excuse to justify a lack of activity. As you look for ways to increase your activity level, keep these tips in mind:

- Choose something that is fun and enjoyable. You will never stick to any activity program if you dread or hate it.

- Wear comfortable, well-fitting shoes and socks.

- If you are a type 1 diabetic, you will need to work with your doctor in order to adjust insulin doses while increasing your activity. Realize that exercising will lower your blood sugar; this can be potentially dangerous in a type 1 diabetic.

- The Centers for Disease Control and Prevention recommends brisk walking five days a week for thirty minutes. Start by walking only ten minutes a day and gradually increase your time to thirty minutes.

RECOMMENDED LEVEL OF INTENSITY

Every activity either requires or can be performed at different levels of intensity. Given that, it makes sense that every person hoping to lose weight has an ideal intensity at which he or she should work out. This is called your target heart rate zone, which generally ranges from 65 to 85 percent of your maximum heart rate.

To calculate the low end of this zone, start by subtracting your age from 220. This is your maximum heart rate. For example, for someone forty years old the formula is:

$$220 - 40 = 180 \text{ beats per minute}$$

Multiply this number by 65 percent to find the low end of the target heart rate zone:

$$180 \times 0.65 = 117 \text{ beats per minute}$$

To figure out the high end of the zone, multiply maximum heart rate by 85 percent:

$$180 \times 0.85 = 153 \text{ beats per minute}$$

So, if you are forty, you should keep your heart rate between 117 and 153 beats per minute when exercising.

High-intensity aerobic exercise actually decreases insulin levels and increases levels of glucagon. By lowering insulin levels, you begin to release more stored body fat, and thus you burn fat, not carbohydrates. I recommend that you maintain a moderate pace as you exercise to keep your body burning fat as fuel.

When you exercise to the point that you are severely short of breath, you are no longer performing aerobically. Instead you have shifted to an anaerobic activity, which burns glycogen—stored sugar—as primary fuel instead of fat. I will explain the benefits of anaerobic activity a little later in this chapter. If you are just starting to exercise and aim to burn primarily fat, you need to work out at a moderate intensity of 65 to 85 percent of your maximum heart rate. This is the fat-burning range of your target heart rate zone.

When you start any activity program, I recommend you work out at around 65 percent of your maximum heart rate. As you become more aerobically conditioned, gradually increase the intensity to 70 percent of maximum heart rate. After a few more weeks, increase to 75 percent, and so on. You may never be able to work out at 85 percent of maximum rate, especially if you are huffing and puffing. Be sure that as you increase the intensity of your workouts, you remain able to converse with another person.

MUSCLES AND METABOLISM

Have you thought that having a high metabolism was others' blessing but not yours? It can be. Your metabolic rate is dependent upon your muscle mass. The more muscle mass you have, the higher your metabolic rate. If your dieting efforts do not include exercise, you can begin to burn muscle mass to supply your body with amino acids and sabotage your weight-loss efforts by slowing down your metabolic rate. The body will then begin to burn fewer calories and less fat. The more muscle you carry, the higher the metabolic rate and the more stored body fat you will burn—even at rest.

THE BENEFITS OF ANAEROBIC EXERCISE

Anaerobic exercise such as weightlifting, sprinting, and resistance training will help to increase lean muscle mass—thereby increasing your metabolic rate. If the workout is intense enough, growth hormone will be released from the pituitary gland. This leads to increased muscle growth and increased fat loss.

For maximum results, however, the exercise must be very strenuous and done until muscle exhaustion occurs or until you simply cannot move any more. This stimulates the release of a powerful surge of growth hormone, which helps to repair and rebuild the muscles that have been broken down during the workout. As you gain more muscle mass, your metabolic rate rises.

A word of caution, however: if you weigh yourself, the scale may not show a dramatic weight loss since the muscle mass that you are adding actually weighs more than the fat it is replacing.

I encourage my patients not to begin resistance training until they are in the routine of walking approximately thirty minutes five days a week. If you are just beginning a weight-lifting program, I recommend that you consult a certified personal trainer who will develop a well-rounded weight-lifting program for you.

As you exercise, be sure to maintain proper form and lift the weights slowly to avoid injury. You should typically perform ten to twelve repetitions per set. When starting resistance training, I recommend only performing one set per activity to reduce soreness. As you become better conditioned over time, you can increase to two or three sets per activity.

Increased sugar and increased starch will inhibit growth hormone release and is counterproductive. Therefore, prior to a workout, avoid snacks that are high in sugar or carbohydrates since you will not have the advantage of this powerful hormone for fat loss and muscle gain.

> He restores my soul; He leads me in the paths of righteousness for His name's sake.
>
> —PSALM 23:3, NKJV

High-intensity interval training (HIIT) can also be an effective anaerobic workout. HIIT is simply alternating between brief, hard bursts of exercise and short stretches of lower-intensity exercise or rest, usually for a period of less than twenty minutes. Various studies in recent years have proven this to be an effective way to improve not only overall cardiovascular health but also your ability to burn fat faster. One study at the University of Guelph in Ontario, Canada, found that following an interval training session with an hour of moderate cycling increased the amount of fat burned by 36 percent.[1]

I personally do HIIT three times a week. I warm up on the elliptical machine for five to ten minutes. I then do sixty seconds of high-intensity training with high resistance and as fast as I can. I then decrease the resistance and speed to a lower setting for one minute. I continue this pattern for twenty minutes or more.

High-intensity anaerobic workouts obviously have proven value.

However, I suggest that you hold off on HIIT, regardless of your exercise past, until you've consistently done some moderate-intensity activity for several months. I'd rather see you be able to sustain your momentum for the long haul rather than have you burn out, not because of eating the wrong things, but simply because you wanted to sprint to the finish line faster. Be sure to have a physical exam with EKG and or a stress test before starting HIIT.

A **BIBLE CURE** *Health Tip*

The Tabata Method

A popular new form of HIIT is Tabata, an exercise regimen created by Izumi Tabata that uses twenty seconds of high-intensity exercise followed by ten seconds of rest, repeated for eight cycles. An alternative routine uses three minutes of warming up, followed by sixty seconds of high-intensity exercise, followed by seventy-five seconds of rest, repeated for eight to twelve cycles.

HOW MUCH EXERCISE IS ENOUGH?

The Centers for Disease Control and Prevention (CDC) and the National Institutes of Health (NIH) recommend that adults need to participate in two categories of physical activity weekly—aerobic exercises and muscle-strengthening exercises. For aerobic activity they recommend two hours and thirty minutes of moderate intensity aerobic activity (brisk walking, water aerobics, riding a bike on level ground, playing doubles tennis, pushing a lawn mower, etc.) every week, or one hour and fifteen minutes of vigorous exercise (jogging, swimming laps, riding a bike fast or on hills/inclines, playing singles tennis, playing basketball, etc.) every week. For muscle-strengthening exercise, which I call resistance exercise, they recommend working all major muscle groups (abdomen, arms, back, chest, hips, legs, and shoulders) two or more days a week.[2]

I recommend breaking up the aerobic activity as follows: if you can only do moderate intensity activities, try brisk walking for thirty minutes a day, five days a week. If you can handle more vigorous activity, jog for twenty-five minutes a day, three days a week. Or you can break it down even further: try going for a ten-minute walk, three times a day, five days a week.

MONITOR YOURSELF

I believe in monitoring yourself. An excellent way to monitor the steps you walk during the day is by using a pedometer. Typically a person walks three thousand to five thousand steps a day. To stay fit, set a goal of ten thousand steps, or approximately five miles. To lose weight, aim for between twelve thousand and fifteen thousand steps per day.

Before engaging in any activity, make sure that you have either eaten a meal two or three hours prior or have had a healthy snack about thirty to sixty minutes beforehand. It is never good to work out when hungry; you may end up burning muscle protein as energy—which is very expensive fuel. Remember, losing muscle lowers your metabolic rate.

> For He satisfies the longing soul, and fills the hungry soul with goodness.
> —PSALM 107:9, NKJV

THE IMPORTANCE OF SLEEP

Getting a good's night sleep is another way to stimulate release of growth hormone in order to build muscle. Growth hormone is secreted during the first couple of hours of sleep, which is stage three and stage four sleep.

HITTING A PLATEAU

If you lose weight steadily and then seem to hit a plateau, exercise will help. By increasing the frequency and duration of exercise, you can break through that plateau and continue losing weight. Try to increase your exercise time gradually from thirty minutes to forty-five minutes. Those stubborn last few pounds will soon begin to melt away.

STEWARDING THE GIFT OF YOUR BODY

Your body is a tremendous gift. With God's help you can feel better and look amazing as you get into shape. Decide right now to begin putting these exercise tips into practice and then, most importantly, to stay with it. Remember, everyone falls down, but it takes an individual with courage to get back up again. You will have your ups and downs—we all do. But hang in there. As I said, stay with it, and before you know it, you will look like the person you've always wanted to become!

A **BIBLE CURE** *Prayer for You*

Lord, I surrender all my cares to You. Give me the power of a disciplined life. Thank You for the gift of my body. I realize that it is a temple of the Holy Spirit and I must be a good steward of it. Each time I become discouraged or want to quit, please be there to pick me up and put me back on track. I surrender the care of my body to You and Your wonderful wisdom. In the name of Jesus Christ, amen.

A **BIBLE CURE** *Prescription*

Check the lifestyle changes you are willing to make to achieve weight loss:

❏ Exercise regularly. The type of exercise you will choose is:

_____

_____

_____

❏ Get enough sleep.

❏ Begin a strengthening program.

❏ Other: _____

Write a prayer asking God for help in making these lifestyle changes.

_____

_____

_____

Write a prayer of commitment asking God for His help in staying faithful to an exercise program. Also, ask your spouse or a friend to exercise with you. An accountability partner increases the success of any weight loss program.

_____

_____

_____

_____

_____

_____

_____

Chapter 7

SUPPLEMENTS THAT SUPPORT WEIGHT LOSS

Your body is the temple of God's Spirit. The apostle Paul writes, "Do you not know that your body is the temple of the Holy Spirit who is in you, whom you have from God, and you are not your own? For you were bought at a price; therefore glorify God in your body and in your spirit, which are God's" (1 Cor. 6:19–20, NKJV).

Your body is also the most incredible creation in the entire universe. All the money in the world could not replace it. It's God's awesome gift and a suitable place to house His own Spirit. Since your body was created as the temple of God's Spirit, it's important to understand that you and I are merely stewards of this gift God has given us.

If you went out today and purchased a Mercedes-Benz or a Porsche, no doubt you would polish it and fill it with the best gas and the best oil—treating it with the respect that such a fine machine deserves. You can honor God in your body as well by treating it with the respect and care that befits such a wonderful gift.

By giving your body the nutrients, vitamins, and minerals it needs to function at peak performance, you will bring honor to God by properly caring for your body—the temple He created on earth to house His own Spirit.

WHAT IS YOUR BODY TRYING TO TELL YOU?

Your incredible body is so sophisticated that it is programmed to signal you that it needs a nutrient or a vitamin you haven't supplied. These signals come in the form of cravings. Have you ever just had to have a glass of orange juice? Your body was probably telling your brain that it needed more vitamin C.

> But those who wait on the LORD shall renew their strength; they shall mount up with wings like eagles, they shall run and not be weary, they shall walk and not faint.
>
> —ISAIAH 40:31, NKJV

Cravings can come following a meal when the body realizes that, although it's been fed, it still hasn't received enough of the nutrients it expected. Too often, instead of discerning the craving properly, we simply fuel our bodies with even more nonnutritious food. Therefore the cravings return, and we respond once again with more junk food. The cycle becomes vicious, we get fatter, and our bodies suffer for lack of real nutrition.

If you experience such cravings, it's likely your body is actually slightly malnourished. Vitamins, minerals, and supplements are vital in today's world for the proper fueling of our bodies. You see, most old-time farmers know that in order for soil to supply the food it produces with a rich supply of vitamins and minerals, it must rest or lie fallow. In other words, it must remain unused every few years. In today's world of high-tech agriculture, this no longer occurs. Therefore our food supplies are actually depleted of the vitamins, minerals, and nutrients our bodies need to maintain good health. So we give our bodies more and more food, but they still lack vitamins and nutrients. That's where supplementation can bridge the gap.

NATURAL SUBSTANCES FOR YOU

Let's explore some of these natural substances that can promote health and vitality as you defeat obesity in your life. Since there are many causes of obesity, I recommend safe nutritional supplements that work through different mechanisms, such as thermogenic agents, natural appetite suppressants that increase satiety, supplements that increase insulin sensitivity, and energy products. We will also look at some of the supplements available that you should avoid as you take the necessary steps to reach your ideal weight.

Vitamins and minerals

A good multivitamin and multimineral. It's important to be sure that you get a good supply of all the various vitamins your body needs, especially if it is depleted. Most multivitamins contain only twelve vitamins in their inactive form. You may want to choose a multivitamin you can take two to three times a day. To prevent our adrenal glands from becoming exhausted, we need to supplement our diets daily with a comprehensive multivitamin and mineral formula with adequate amounts of B-complex vitamins. Divine Health Active Multivitamin has the active form of the vitamins, chelated minerals, and antioxidants in a balanced comprehensive formula.

Choosing a mineral supplement is a little more difficult than choosing a vitamin supplement and sometimes more costly. Find a mineral supplement that is chelated rather than one that contains mineral salts. Chelation is a process of wrapping a mineral with an organic molecule such as an amino acid that increases absorption dramatically. (See appendix B.)

Green Supreme Food. This supplement contains fifteen organic fruits, veggies, and superfoods, as well as probiotics, fiber, antioxidants, and phytonutrients. It helps energize, detoxify, and create an alkaline environment in the tissue, helping one lose weight.

Thermogenic (fat-burning) agents

The term *thermogenic* describes the body's natural means of raising its temperature to burn off more calories. More specifically, thermogenesis is the process of triggering the body to burn white body fat, which is the kind of fat we often accumulate as we age. Thermogenic agents, then, are fat burners that help to increase the rate of white-body-fat breakdown. Fortunately, most unsafe thermogenic agents have been pulled off the market.

Green tea. Green tea and green tea extract are good weight-loss supplements. Green tea has been used for thousands of years in Asia as both a tea and an herbal medicine. It has two key ingredients: a catechin called epigallocatechin gallate (EGCG) and caffeine. Both lead to the release of more epinephrine, which then increases the metabolic rate. Ultimately green tea promotes fat oxidation, which is fat burning. It also increases the rate at which you burn calories over a twenty-four-hour period.

An effective daily dose of EGCG is 90 milligrams or more, which can be consumed by drinking three or four cups of green tea a day.

Do not add sugar, honey, or artificial sweeteners to it, though you may use the natural sweetener stevia. In addition to drinking green tea, I recommend 100 milligrams of green tea supplement three times a day. (See appendix B.)

> It is vain for you to rise up early, to sit up late, to eat the bread of sorrows; for so He gives His beloved sleep.
> —PSALM 127:2, NKJV

Green coffee bean extract. In January 2012 a placebo-controlled study reported that every participant experienced weight loss caused by green coffee bean extract. For twenty-two weeks participants were given 350 milligrams of green coffee bean extract twice a day. They did not change their diets, averaging 2,400 calories per day, but they did burn 400 calories a day through exercise. The average weight loss was 17.6 pounds, with some subjects losing 22.7 pounds, and there were no side effects.[1]

The key phytonutrient in green coffee bean extract is chlorogenic acid, which can decrease the uptake of carbohydrates, fats, and glucoses from the intestines and thus decrease calorie absorption. It also has positive effects on how your body processes glucose and fats, and it helps to lower blood sugar and insulin levels. Drinking coffee doesn't give you the same effects. Because of roasting, most of the chlorogenic acid in coffee is destroyed. By comparison, the extract is much better. Green coffee bean extract should contain 45 percent or more of chlorogenic acid. In addition to—or in place of—drinking coffee, I recommend taking 400 milligrams of green coffee bean extract thirty minutes before each meal. (See appendix B.)

Meratrim. Meratrim is a blend of two plant extracts that has been shown to significantly reduce body weight, BMI, and waist measurement within eight weeks when used with a diet and exercise plan. The studies show that 400 milligrams of Meratrim twice a day, thirty minutes before breakfast and thirty minutes before dinner, achieved these results by interfering with the accumulation of fat while simultaneously increasing fat burning.[2] (See appendix B.)

Thyroid support

All obese patients should be screened for hypothyroidism, using tests such as the blood tests TSH, free T3, free T4, and thyroid peroxidase antibodies, to rule out Hashimoto's thyroiditis, the most common cause of low thyroid. If a patient has low body temperature (less than 98 degrees), they most likely have a sluggish metabolism and may have sluggish thyroid function. It's especially important to optimize the free T3 blood level to improve the metabolic rate. The normal range of T3, according to the lab I use, is 2.1 to 4.4. I try to optimize the T3 level to a range of 3.0 to 4.2 by using both levothyroxine (T4) and liothyronine (T3). I can sometimes optimize the T3 levels with natural supplements including Metabolic Advantage or iodine supplements. I also commonly perform a lab test to see if a patient is low in iodine before starting iodine supplements. According to the American Thyroid Association, "Approximately 40 percent of the world's population [is] at risk for iodine deficiency."[3]

Appetite suppressants

These supplements generally act on the central nervous system to decrease appetite or create a sensation of fullness. Although some medications in this category include risk-prone phenylpropanolamine (found in such products as Dexatrim), I have found a few safe, natural supplements that are extremely effective appetite suppressants.

L-tryptophan and 5-HTP. These are amino acids that help the body to manufacture serotonin. Serotonin assists in controlling carbohydrate and sugar cravings. L-tryptophan and 5-HTP also function like natural antidepressants. If you are taking migraine medications called triptans or SSRIs (selective serotonin reuptake inhibitors), you should talk with your physician before taking either supplement. The typical dose of L-tryptophan is 500 to 2,000 milligrams at bedtime. For 5-HTP it is typically 50 to 100 milligrams one to three times a day or 100 to 300 milligrams at bedtime. Serotonin Max is an excellent supplement that helps boost serotonin levels naturally. (See appendix B.)

L-tyrosine, N-acetyl L-tyrosine, and L-phenylalanine. These are naturally occurring amino acids found in numerous protein foods, including cottage cheese, turkey, and chicken. They help to raise norepinephrine and dopamine levels in the brain, which then helps decrease appetite and cravings and improves your mood. Doses of L-tyrosine, N-acetyl L-tyrosine, and L-phenylalanine may range from 500 to 2,000 milligrams a day (sometimes higher), but they should be taken on an empty stomach. I prefer N-acetyl L-tyrosine for most of my patients since the body absorbs it better than L-tyrosine or L-phenylalanine. I typically start patients on 500 to 1,000 milligrams of N-acetyl L-tyrosine, taken thirty minutes before breakfast and thirty minutes before lunch. I do not recommend taking any of these supplements in late afternoon because they may interfere with sleep. (See appendix B.)

Supplements to increase satiety

Fiber supplements and foods high in fiber increase feelings of fullness by using several different mechanisms. Fiber slows the passage of food through the digestive tract, decreases the absorption of sugars and starches into the stomach, and expands and fills up the stomach—turning down the appetite. Although the American Heart Association and the National Cancer Institute recommend 30 grams or more of fiber each day, the average American only consumes between 12 and 17 grams.[4]

When it comes to losing weight and managing blood sugar levels, a little fiber goes a long way. One study found that consuming an extra 14 grams of soluble fiber each day for only two days was associated with a 10 percent decrease in caloric intake.[5] Soluble fiber supplements significantly increase post-meal satisfaction and should be taken before each meal to assist in weight loss. Soluble fiber lowers the blood sugar, slowing down digestion and the absorption of sugars and carbohydrates. This allows for a more gradual rise in blood sugar, which lowers the glycemic index of the foods you eat. This helps to improve the blood sugar levels.

The fiber that I prefer for weight-loss patients is PGX. I start with one capsule, taken with 8 to 16 ounces of water before each meal and snack, and then gradually increase the dose to two to four capsules until patients can control their appetite. Always take PGX with evening meals and snacks.

In addition to PGX, another great fiber for weight loss is

glucomannan, made from the Asian root konjac. Glucomannan is five times more effective in lowering cholesterol when compared to other fibers such as psyllium, oat fiber, or guar gum. Because it expands to ten times its original size when placed in water, it is a great supplement to take before a meal to reduce your appetite as it expands in your stomach, but you should take it with 16 ounces of water or unsweetened black or green tea. (See appendix B.)

Supplements to increase energy production

L-carnitine is an amino acid that helps our bodies turn food into energy by shuttling fatty acids into the mitochondria, which act as our cells' energy factories by burning fatty acids for energy. Humans synthesize very little carnitine, so we may need to supplement from outside sources. This applies especially to obese and older individuals, who typically have lower levels of carnitine than the average-weight segment of the population. As you might expect, individuals with insufficient carnitine have a greater difficulty burning fat for energy.

> For the kingdom of God is not eating and drinking, but righteousness and peace and joy in the Holy Spirit.
> —ROMANS 14:17, NKJV

Milk, meat such as mutton and lamb, fish, and cheese are good sources of L-carnitine. In supplement form, I recommend taking a combination of L-carnitine and acetyl L-carnitine, lipoic acid, PQQ (pyrroloquinoline quinone), and a glutathione-boosting supplement. The best time to take these supplements is in the morning and early afternoon (before 3:00 p.m.) on an empty stomach. If you take them any later, these supplements can impair your sleep. Green tea supplements and N-acetyl L-tyrosine also help to increase your energy.

Other common supplements to assist with weight loss

Irvingia. Irvingia is a fruit-bearing plant grown in the jungles of Cameroon in Africa. Irvingia gabonensis helps to resensitize your cells to insulin. It appears to be able to reverse leptin resistance by lowering levels of C-reactive protein (CRP), an inflammatory mediator. Leptin is a hormone that tells your brain you've eaten enough and that it is time to stop. It also enhances your body's ability to use fat as an energy source. One also needs zinc, 12 to 15 milligrams a day, which is present in most comprehensive multivitamins, in order for leptin to function optimally.

Because of Americans' sedentary lifestyles and highly processed, high-glycemic food choices, many overweight and obese patients have acquired resistance to leptin. As a result, this hormone no longer works properly in their bodies. Similar to insulin resistance, leptin resistance is a chronic inflammatory condition that contributes to weight gain. It is critically important to follow the anti-inflammatory dietary program I have outlined in this book. Simply decreasing inflammatory foods enables most to start losing belly fat and also allows leptin to function optimally. The generally recommended dose is 150 milligrams of standardized Irvingia extract, twice a day, thirty minutes before lunch and dinner.

7-keto-DHEA. Derived from the hormone dehydroepiandrosterone (DHEA), 7-keto-DHEA is taken to help rev a person's metabolism to aid in weight loss. Unlike its "parent hormone" DHEA, which is produced by glands near the kidneys, 7-keto-DHEA does not affect sex hormone levels in the body.[6] The supplement is also used to boost the immune system, build muscle, enhance memory, improve lean body mass, and slow aging, though there is limited scientific evidence to support all of those benefits.[7] However, 7-keto-DHEA has been shown to increase the resting metabolic rate in those who were already dieting and engaging in regular exercise. An eight-week study found that those taking 100 mg of 7-keto-DHEA twice daily lost approximately six pounds while those who received a placebo lost a little over two pounds.[8] The supplement was not found to have any adverse side effects after a series of toxicological evaluations. A safety study published in *Clinical Investigative Medicine* indicated that 7-keto-DHEA was safe for human consumption in doses of 200 mg per day for up to four weeks. The safety of internal use beyond four weeks is not known.[9]

The hoodia controversy. Hoodia is a South African plant similar to a cactus that may help suppress the appetite. Initially used by tribal leaders to enable them to go on long journeys without getting hungry, various sources cite thousands of years' worth of Bushman history to verify its effectiveness. Although these tribal hunters obviously have not conducted scientific studies to prove hoodia is an effective appetite suppressant, one 2001 clinical study by a company called Phytopharm found individuals who consumed the plant ate 1,000 fewer calories a day than those who didn't take hoodia.[10] One of the company's researchers, Richard Dixey, MD, explained that hoodia contains a molecule that is ten thousand times more active than glucose.[11] However, there is a catch. When news of this supposed miracle supplement hit the headlines, dozens (if not hundreds) of companies started marketing hoodia—without having any actual hoodia in their products. The result was that more hoodia was "produced" in a single year than in all of African history—highly unlikely, to say the least. Even today it is possible that much of what is sold in the United States either contains ineffective hoodia variations or no hoodia. So be wary of falling for marketing schemes with this substance.

No Magic Bullet

There is no magic weight-loss pill. Scientists have been searching for "The Pill to End All Diets" for years, and no magic bullet has been found. There have been several attempts, including the popular fen-phen back in the nineties. While individuals lost weight, after only a few years a small percentage of users died of a rare disease called primary pulmonary hypertension. This affected several patients out of one hundred thousand; about half of them eventually required a heart-lung transplant to survive. The drug was eventually pulled, and several years later another miracle cure seemed to emerge. Combining ephedra with caffeine seemed to be a powerful formula for turning down the appetite and burning fat. But in time the safety of ephedra was also called into question. It has been linked with severe side effects, including arrhythmias, heart attack, stroke, hypertension, psychosis, seizure, and even death.

Due to safety concerns, in 2004 the Food and Drug Administration (FDA) banned ephedra products in the United States. Although a federal court later upheld the ban, companies wiggle around it by selling extracts that contain little or no ephedrine. And some related herbs, such as bitter orange (citrus aurantium) and country mallow, remain on the market. Like ephedra, bitter orange supplements have been linked to stroke, cardiac arrest, angina, heart attack, ventricular arrhythmias, and death. These products are potentially lethal. I do not recommend them unless taken under the direction and close monitoring of a knowledgeable physician.

A **BIBLE CURE** Health Fact

Alli and Hydroxycut Side Effects

Alli, one of the most common over-the-counter diet pills, may cause bowel changes in its users. These changes, which result from undigested fat going through the digestive system, may include gas with an oily discharge, loose stools or diarrhea, more frequent and urgent bowel movements, and hard-to-control bowel movements. Hydroxycut products were recalled in May 2009 after reports of deadly liver failure and disease in individuals who took the products to lose weight. According to the *World Journal of Gastroenterology*, an ingredient in Hydroxycut from a fruit called Garcinia cambogia caused the liver disease and failure.[12]

Among other herbs of concern is aristolochia, which is found in some Chinese herbal weight-loss supplements and may not even be listed as an ingredient. Aristolochia is a known kidney toxin and carcinogen in humans. There are also products containing usnea (usnic acid), a lichen for weight loss that can cause severe liver toxicity. In addition, some Brazilian diet pills have been found to be contaminated with amphetamines and other prescription drugs.[13]

A weight-loss supplement is a nutritional product or herb intended to assist your healthy eating and activity plan with the ultimate goal of losing weight. A supplement comes alongside; it does not replace. Do not be deceived by crafty marketing that promises otherwise. Weight-loss and dietary supplements are not subject to the same standards as prescription drugs or medications sold over the counter. They can be marketed with only limited proof of safety or effectiveness.

> Therefore, if anyone is in Christ, he is a new creation; old things
> have passed away; behold, all things have become new.
> —2 CORINTHIANS 5:17, NKJV

A LIFESTYLE CHOICE

While some questionable products are on the market, there are a variety of safe, effective over-the-counter dietary supplements for weight loss. Some people may find that incorporating a combination of these into their eating and activity plan works even better. Others may not need to take any supplements. Most of my overweight and obese patients have found that taking a combination of green tea extract, green coffee bean extract, and Irvingia (see appendix B) along with certain amino acids (such as Serotonin Max and N-acetyl L-tyrosine), and PGX fiber supplements before each meal and snack (especially in the evening) helped them shed pounds and controlled their appetites. (See appendix B.)

If you continue experiencing problems controlling your appetite or struggle with food cravings, decreased energy, or insulin resistance, you will likely require one or more of the supplements I just reviewed. The same goes if you do not feel full or satisfied after a meal or if you have low hormone levels.

However, I remind you that supplements are just that—supplements, not magic pills. The truth is that there is no shortcut to losing weight and keeping it off. A new lifestyle that includes good nutrition, exercise, supplementation, and constant diligence is the best way to overcome obesity. The vitamins and supplements I have suggested can help you, but only you can decide to begin an entirely new lifestyle filled with health, vitality, and God's very best! Make that determination at this very moment.

A **BIBLE CURE** Prayer for You

Lord, thank You for vitamins and supplements that can help me battle obesity. Help me to be diligent in a plan to overcome obesity and to live a healthy lifestyle guided by Your Spirit and plan for divine health. Amen.

A **BIBLE CURE** Prescription

Check the steps you are willing to take:

❏ Take a multivitamin.
❏ Drink green tea or take green tea extract.
❏ Use fiber.
❏ Take green coffee bean extract.
❏ Other:

Describe the diligent ways you are living in divine health:

_____

_____

_____

_____

_____

_____

_____

_____

_____

_____

_____

_____

_____

Chapter 8

POWER FOR CHANGE THROUGH FAITH IN GOD

THERE IS NO greater love in the universe than the love God feels for you. No matter what you've done or neglected to do, He loves you more than you could ever know. And He longs to reveal His love to you in every place of emotional need. He tenderly calls you—even now—asking you to give Him all of the hurts, hidden pain, and disappointments that you've been carrying around with you. The Bible instructs us, "Casting all your care upon Him, for He cares about you" (1 Pet. 5:7, NKJV).

Look at what Jesus said in Matthew 11:28: "Come to Me" (NKJV). How often have you—for lack of comfort, nervousness, because of a numb inability to really face your emotional pain, or from a hollow sense of aloneness—opened up the refrigerator and filled an empty place in your heart with a piece of pie or a cupcake?

You see, just as with a drug, food can temporarily anesthetize you from the pain of loneliness, abandonment, fear, stress, and emotional pain. It's no wonder the American population is getting larger. We are a nation emotionally hurting from a lack of love. But food cannot truly fill that void—even if we haven't faced it for so long that we hardly notice it anymore.

> Being confident of this very thing, that He who has begun a good work in you will complete it until the day of Jesus Christ.
> —PHILIPPIANS 1:6, NKJV

But I have really good news for you. Jesus Christ can fill it, and He can comfort your heart with a sense of peace that will overwhelm you with true joy.

You see, Jesus Christ died for you in order to meet your need and comfort your pain. And He is just as alive today and as real as when He walked the shores of Galilee. Make the choice to let Him tenderly love you. All you need to do is ask Him. His love is just the whisper of a prayer away.

Feeling Guilty About Food Cravings?

Have you ever felt that your cravings for certain foods were somehow a guilty reflection upon you? Unhealthy food cravings are merely your body's way of signaling you that something is out of whack. From now on, commit your cravings to God at the moment they occur. He will give you the strength to get through them without overeating and the grace and wisdom to understand what your body or heart is trying to tell you. Let your cravings begin a process of bringing your body back into physical and spiritual balance, and with that balance, better health. One of the main emotional motivators that can send you racing to the refrigerator for comfort is stress. Stress works against you in other ways too.

Stress Can Make You Fat

The excessive stress you are under on a daily basis can contribute to obesity. When you are under stress, your body produces a hormone called cortisol, which is very similar to cortisone. If you have ever taken cortisone, you are well aware of the side effects. Cortisone causes you to gain weight.

Cortisol can have the same effect. When your adrenal glands produce cortisol during periods of high anxiety and stress, it can actually cause your body to gain weight. Therefore reducing your level of stress can help you lose weight and keep it off.

A Closer Look

Stress affects the heart, the blood vessels, and the immune system, but it also directly affects our adrenal glands. The adrenal glands, along with the thyroid gland, help to maintain the body's energy levels. God's plan for your life will help you to lower your stress. His plan for you is good and not bad. "For I know the thoughts that I think toward you, says the LORD, thoughts of peace and not of evil, to give you a future and a hope. Then you will call upon Me and go and pray to Me, and I will listen to you. And you will seek Me and find Me, when you search for Me with all your heart" (Jer. 29:11–13, NKJV).

THE POWER OF SCRIPTURE

God wants you to surrender your cares to Him and allow His peace to rule in your heart. Memorize and meditate on these two promises for your life:

> Be anxious for nothing, but in everything by prayer and supplication, with thanksgiving, let your requests be made known to God; and the peace of God, which surpasses all understanding, will guard your hearts and minds through Christ Jesus.
>
> —PHILIPPIANS 4:6–7 , NKJV

> Casting all your care upon Him, for He cares for you.
>
> —1 PETER 5:7, NKJV

When you hold on to your worries and cares, you find yourself under stress and overeating or not watching what you eat. When you are depressed and believing the worst is yet to come, you may try to use food as comfort. Trust God's Word and plan for your life, and turn all your cares and worries over to Him.

THE COMFORTER IS COME

God knows how tough our lives can be and how often we face life's difficulties alone. That's why He provided Himself as our Comforter. When the light goes on inside of your heart, when you really understand that God is real, that He is alive, that you are not alone, and that He is able to provide you the comfort you need, you will never reach for the empty comfort of food again. I encourage you to study the scriptures throughout this Bible Cure; read them over and over again. At the moment you are tempted to reach for comfort from food, read a verse and pray. God is able to give you the strength and help you need to overcome any and all emotional aspects of obesity. He will set you completely free.

THE BREAD OF LIFE

Jesus says that He is the bread of life. When you feel emotional cravings for sweets, carbohydrates, and other foods that you do not need, turn to the bread that you need—Jesus Christ. Let your cravings for rich food be transformed into signals that turn you to true riches in Christ. Remember His words:

> I am the bread of life. He who comes to Me shall never hunger, and he who believes in Me shall never thirst.
> —JOHN 6:35, NKJV

As you've read through this book, I hope you've discovered that although God is very powerful, He came to share His power with you. You are not powerless in the face of temptation, fear, loneliness, or confusion. One of the most wonderful things about Jesus Christ is that He is very near. Reach out to Him for all of your needs. You will not be disappointed.

A BIBLE CURE Prayer for You

Lord God, You alone are my strength and my source. My ability to stay committed to weight loss and healthy eating comes from You. Help me maintain the willpower I need. Give me the focus I need to implement all that I am learning. Almighty God, replace any discouragement with hope and any doubt with faith. I know that You are with me and will not leave me. I thank You, Lord, for seeing me through this battle and giving me victory over obesity. Amen.

A **BIBLE CURE** *Prescription*

This is a daily checklist to copy and keep on your refrigerator, in your purse, or in your briefcase. Do each one daily for best results.

❏ I awakened and confessed that this body belongs to Jesus, and I'll give my body what it needs and not what it craves.

❏ I can do all things through Christ who strengthens me, and that includes losing weight.

❏ I thanked God throughout the day that I am slender and energetic, my health is restored, and my strength is renewed. (You may not be slender now, but start saying it by faith.)

❏ I ate a balanced breakfast, lunch, dinner, and snack according to the Bible Cure plan.

❏ I determined to walk in faith today with God's help.

❏ I took vitamins and supplements according to the Bible Cure plan. I exercised according to the Bible Cure plan.

❏ I feel strong and disciplined with God's help.

❏ I thank God throughout the day because now losing weight is easy for me.

THE BIBLE CURE
FOR THYROID DISORDERS

Chapter 9

DO YOU HAVE A HIDDEN PROBLEM?

EELING REALLY TIRED lately? Perhaps you've gained weight or just can't seem to lose it no matter how hard you try. Are you cold all the time? Is your skin dryer than usual, or have you noticed that you seem extra thirsty or just achy? Maybe you've been kind of down, forgetful, constipated or unusually irritable. If any of these sound like you, you may be a part of a hidden epidemic: *hypothyroidism* or *low-thyroid function*.

If so, it's no accident that you've picked up this Bible Cure book. For God's Word declares that He works to bring hidden things to light. Luke 12:2 says, "But there is nothing covered up that will not be revealed, and hidden that will not be known" (NASB).

It's estimated that more than 13 million American women have some kind of thyroid dysfunction, and many of them do not know it. Men have it, too.[1]

Thyroid disorders hide in the darkness of our ignorance, far from view, which allows them to wreak havoc with our health and peace of mind. They are one of the most underdiagnosed problems today, and professionals easily miss many of their symptoms. In fact, experts estimate that more than half of those with low-grade hypothyroidism remain undiagnosed. Researchers say about 10 percent of younger women and 20 percent of women over fifty regularly experience mild thyroid problems that impact their weight, attitude and overall health.[2] As we will see, milder cases of thyroid disorder often do not show up in standard medical tests, yet they still create distressing symptoms.

Sadly, for the millions suffering from a thyroid disorder of which they are entirely unaware, the Bible says in Hosea 4:6, "My people are destroyed for lack of knowledge" (NASB). These individuals could be unknowingly harming their bodies by not eating the right foods or taking the right supplements or medications.

Nevertheless, I have good news for you. God wants you well and happy, and He is at work to bring hidden problems to light in order to heal them for you. In fact, He has wonderful plans for your life! He has a purpose for you—a special task on this earth only you can fulfill. The Bible clearly declares that God wishes above all things that you prosper and be in health, even as your soul prospers (3 John 2, NKJV). God's wonderful plan for your life includes terrific, vibrant health.

Unfortunately, there is a devil who would like nothing more than to see you unable to fulfill your destiny. Jesus promised to give us life and life more abundantly. He also said that the purpose of the devil is to kill, steal and destroy (John 10:10). Your adversary will use every trick in the book to keep you down and defeated—and that includes bringing hidden sickness and disease upon your body. But God has revealed the wisdom we need through the field of medicine, natural remedies He has placed on this earth and, most powerfully, His mighty Word and healing power.

SPIRITUAL ROOTS OF DISEASE

As a Christian medical doctor, I have studied and prayed about the causes of disease for many years. Increasingly, I have discovered that many diseases have strong spiritual roots. God is interested in the health of the entire person—body, mind and spirit. Although traditional medicine often sees these facets of our being as separate, in truth they are not. A vital link exists between the spirit, soul and body. That's why this Bible Cure is strategically designed to bring God's healing power to your heart, mind and spirit through the power of faith and God's wonderful Word.

No matter what the cause is of your thyroid condition, with His help and with the truths you will learn from this book, you *will* overcome. This Bible Cure book is filled with hope and encouragement for understanding how to keep your body fit and in a healthy balance. In it you will

*uncover God's divine plan of health for body, soul and
spirit through modern medicine, good nutrition and
the medicinal power of Scripture and prayer.*

You will find key Scripture passages throughout this book that will help you focus on the power of God. These divine promises will empower your prayers and redirect your thoughts to line up with God's plan of divine health for you—a plan that includes victory over whatever thyroid condition may be afflicting you.

This Bible Cure book will give you a strategic plan for divine health, covering topics such as lifestyle factors, supplements, nutrition, and faith.

If you are suffering from a thyroid disorder, take fresh confidence in the knowledge that God is real. He is alive, and He loves you more than you could ever imagine. You *will* enjoy complete restoration of your health—body, mind and spirit.

It is my prayer that these powerful godly insights will bring health, wholeness and spiritual refreshing to you. May they deepen your fellowship with God and strengthen your ability to worship and serve Him, fulfilling your divine purpose on the earth.

A **BIBLE CURE** *Prayer for You*

*Heavenly Father, I pray that You will help apply the truths
from this book as I trust You to help me with my thyroid disorders. Let Your wisdom guide me as I allow Your healing
power to come to my body, mind and spirit through the
power of faith and Your Word. In Jesus' name, amen.*

Chapter 10

A LAMP OF UNDERSTANDING

THE PRESENCE OF God in your life is a constantly burning flame of wisdom, power, knowledge, peace and help. If you let Him, He will light a pathway to total restoration and radiant refreshing. In fact, the Bible says, "Your word is a lamp to guide my feet and a light for my path" (Ps. 119:105, NLT).

The first step along your pathway is wisdom and understanding. "Joyful is the person who finds wisdom, the one who gains understanding.... Wisdom is a tree of life to those who embrace her" (Prov. 3:13, 18, NLT). You may wonder, *How do I get this wisdom?* It's really not complicated. The Bible says simply go out and get it.

Therefore, let's begin this Bible Cure by taking the first step: gaining a good understanding of the thyroid and its disorders. In this chapter you will discover whether you may have a thyroid disorder and what it means if you do.

> Let all that I am praise the LORD; may I never forget the good things he does for me. He forgives all my sins and heals all my diseases.
>
> —PSALM 103:2–3, NLT

YOUR THYROID

Until a problem occurs, most people never consider their thyroid gland or how important it is to the health of their bodies. The thyroid actually has a shape similar to a butterfly, with two lobes that extend like wings. They stretch across the front of the lower part of your neck, straddling your windpipe between your breastbone and Adam's apple.

WHAT YOU SHOULD KNOW

The main purpose of the thyroid gland is to produce and release two hormones that are vitally important to your body: T3 (or triiodothyronine) and T4 (or thyroxine).

The signal for thyroid hormone production actually begins in the brain. The part of the brain called the *hypothalamus* produces a hormone called TRH (thyrotropin-releasing hormone). This hormone is sent to the pituitary gland beneath the hypothalamus, which triggers it to release TSH (thyroid-stimulating hormone). The TSH leaves the pituitary gland and travels in the bloodstream to the thyroid, eventually causing the production and release of the thyroid hormones T3 and T4.

The delicate balance of these hormones makes a great difference to your health. When your body receives too little of these hormones, you will experience *hypothyroidism*, a disease process caused by an *underactive* thyroid gland. Hormones dramatically affect many of the body's systems and functions. That's why low levels of these vital hormones can create a wide range of problems; they impact nearly everything your body tries to do. That includes breaking down fat, regulating menstrual periods and controlling body temperature. With an underactive thyroid, you might experience a weight gain that seems impossible to lose no matter how hard you try.

Hyperthyroidism, just the opposite condition, is caused by an *overactive* thyroid gland. In other words, your body gets too much of these vital hormones, causing you to lose weight, sweat a lot, feel hot when others are comfortable and have a rapid heart rate. Nevertheless, it's still possible to have one of these conditions and experience absolutely no symptoms at all, which is part of the hidden nature of this problem.

Let's examine the symptoms of thyroid disorder a little more closely to help you determine whether or not some of your symptoms are being caused by thyroid hormone imbalance.

WHEN YOUR BODY ATTACKS ITSELF

In the United States as well as in Europe, the primary cause of hypothyroidism is an autoimmune thyroid disease called Hashimoto's thyroiditis. Here your immune system begins attacking your own thyroid gland as if it were a threatening invader. Over time, the thyroid becomes damaged, eventually resulting in hypothyroidism.

A **BIBLE CURE** Health Fact

Do You Have Symptoms?

Answer the following questions to determine if you could have symptoms of an underactive thyroid gland:

- ❑ Do you have unexplained fatigue?
- ❑ Are you weak?
- ❑ Are you lethargic?
- ❑ Are you experiencing unwanted weight gain?
- ❑ Do you have dry skin? Flaky skin?
- ❑ Are you experiencing hair loss?
- ❑ Are you more irritable lately?
- ❑ Are you constipated?
- ❑ Are your hands and feet cold?
- ❑ Are you depressed?
- ❑ Do you have problems concentrating?
- ❑ Are you having irregular menstrual cycles?
- ❑ Do you forget people's names easily?
- ❑ Do you have puffiness and swelling around the eyes, face, feet or hands?
- ❑ Has your voice become hoarse?
- ❑ Are you unable to lose weight with proper diet and exercise?
- ❑ Do you have a history of miscarriages?

In the quiz above, no single question points to a thyroid disorder, but if you answered yes to several of these questions, it is quite possible that you may be suffering from a thyroid imbalance. I strongly recommend that you have your thyroid gland checked by a medical professional who can draw a blood test for TSH and free T4 levels. Also, take this questionnaire to your doctor to more thoroughly discuss your symptoms with him.

Some of the more common symptoms of hypothyroidism are listed in the previous Bible Cure Health Fact, but one unexpected symptom is the thinning of the hair, especially if the hair becomes more brittle and breaks easily, or if you lose the hair in the outer third of your eyebrows.

Many individuals with hypothyroidism experience some degree of depression. A decreased sex drive, infertility, problems achieving pregnancy, menstrual cycle irregularities and an increased risk of miscarriage are also fairly common and unfortunate characteristics of hypothyroidism.

Other symptoms include irritability, muscle weakness, swelling in the neck, brittle nails, elevated cholesterol levels and achy joints. Yet, we've seen that some people have no symptoms at all, which is why it's so important for you to get tested.

HIDE AND SEEK

OK, you say you've been to the doctor and had your thyroid tested, and the results came back as normal. Still you continue to experience a number of symptoms associated with thyroid problems. Before you decide that you have become a hypochondriac, consider this: thyroid levels can fluctuate, and thyroid disease can turn itself on and off. It works a little like the appliance that you finally take to the repair shop, only to find that when the repairman plugs it in it works just fine.

> But he was pierced for our rebellion, crushed for our sins. He was beaten so that we could be whole. He was whipped so we could be healed.
>
> —ISAIAH 53:5, NLT

Just because you've received a clean bill of health following a blood test does not mean you're home free. You may still have a slight thyroid condition that is not showing up in the blood tests, or your hormone levels may simply be a little off balance temporarily. The results are the same: you feel tired, gain weight or experience any of the many other symptoms of thyroid dysfunction.

More experts are realizing that slight fluctuations in thyroid hormones—problems that often do not show up in medical tests—are creating the same distressing symptoms for millions of people.

Women who are experiencing the normal hormonal fluctuations that accompany menopause and peri- or premenopause may experience low thyroid. Low thyroid is the suspected culprit in a host of underlying symptoms of menopause that often go undiagnosed. In fact, by age fifty, one in every twelve women has a significant degree of hypothyroidism. By age sixty, it is one woman out of every six.[1]

A **BIBLE CURE** Health Tip

Get a Checkup!

The American Thyroid Association recommends that serum TSH screening be instituted at age thirty-five in both men and women and be repeated every five years.[2]

GETTING AN ACCURATE DIAGNOSIS

During medical school and throughout my residency, I began to notice that some individuals who had normal TSH levels continued to experience many symptoms of low thyroid. The TSH test is the main blood test to diagnose and manage hypothyroidism.

A normal TSH is considered to be in the range of 0.5 to 5 microunits per milliliter. Yet, today the American Association of Clinical Endocrinologists (AACE) now says that a TSH level between 3.0 and 5.0 microunits per milliliter should be considered representative of hypothyroidism. Despite this official change, many doctors have patients whose TSH levels are between 3 and 5 and who are displaying symptoms of hypothyroidism, yet they continue to dismiss the diagnosis of thyroid disease. The higher the TSH test, the more hypothyroid you are.

SCREEN YOURSELF TO BE SURE

If you suspect your thyroid may be acting up, here's a simple test you can give yourself at home to let you know whether you may have a sluggish thyroid condition.

A **BIBLE CURE** *Health Tip*

Track Your Basal Body Temperature

Some doctors believe that blood tests may not be sensitive enough to detect milder forms of hypothyroidism. This test is easy and is a great indicator of a milder or intermittent form of thyroid dysfunction. I suggest you try it even if you're in doubt. Simply follow these steps:

1. Place a thermometer next to your night stand, but shake it down first to be sure it registers below 95 degrees Fahrenheit. Be sure you can reach it easily without getting out of bed.

2. The following morning before you rise, take your temperature by placing the thermometer under your armpit for ten minutes. Remain as still as possible.

3. Record your temperature reading for at least three consecutive days.

Women should do this during the first two weeks of their menstrual cycle to get an accurate reading. The first day of the menstrual period is the first day of the menstrual cycle.

Normal basal body temperatures fall between 97.4 and 98.2 degrees Fahrenheit. If your reading is consistently below 97.4, you could be hypothyroid.

Many individuals have consistently low basal body temperatures and experience many of the symptoms of hypothyroidism. Yet their thyroid blood tests are normal. For these individuals I recommend further blood tests, including thyroid autoantibodies.

THE OTHER EXTREME: HYPERTHYROIDISM

We have seen what happens when the body doesn't get enough thyroid hormone, but you may be wondering what happens if it gets too much. This thyroid disease is called *hyperthyroidism*. It is far less common, affecting about 2 million Americans, compared to the 11 million suffering with an underactive thyroid.

Hyperthyroidism works much the opposite of hypothyroidism. Where hypothyroidism seems to slow down the body's metabolism, hyperthyroidism revs it up. A thyroid on high throttle can cause very distressing symptoms. Take the test below to see if you may be experiencing hyperthyroidism.

A **BIBLE CURE** Health Fact

Symptoms of Hyperthyroidism

Answer the following questions to determine if you could have symptoms of an overactive thyroid gland:

- ❏ Do you have a rapid or irregular heartbeat?
- ❏ Do you feel nervous much of the time?
- ❏ Are you more irritable?
- ❏ Do your hands shake with tremors?
- ❏ Are you always hungry?
- ❏ Have you lost weight?
- ❏ Do you have a wide-eyed stare?
- ❏ Have you experienced more diarrhea?
- ❏ Do you have menstrual periods with scant bleeding?
- ❏ Are you infertile?
- ❏ Do you sweat a lot when others seem to be comfortable?
- ❏ Are you intolerant to heat?

❑ Do you tire quickly?

❑ Are your muscles weak?

❑ Are you having trouble sleeping?

❑ Are you experiencing mood swings?

❑ Are you experiencing shortness of breath?

❑ Is your hair fine and straight?

❑ Is it sometimes difficult to catch your breath?

Because thyroid disorder can hide from even the best medical examiners, no single symptom points to it. But if you answered yes to several of these symptoms, please get examined by your medical doctor or endocrinologist for hyperthyroidism. Remember that your thyroid helps your body to perform many vital functions, so never take a possible problem lightly.

WHAT YOU NEED TO KNOW

Women are ten times more likely than men to develop hyperthyroidism.[3] The most common cause of hyperthyroidism is Graves' disease, an autoimmune disorder that may cause the thyroid gland to enlarge, usually forming what is known as a goiter. Other causes include an inflammation of the thyroid triggered by a viral infection or childbirth, or the formation of localized lumps or nodules in the gland itself that can cause it to produce too much thyroid hormone. Eating too much iodine may create the same effect; benign and malignant tumors can, too.

> My child, pay attention to what I say. Listen carefully to my words. Don't lose sight of them. Let them penetrate deep into your heart, for they bring life to those who find them, and healing to their whole body.
>
> —PROVERBS 4:20–22, NLT

Dr. Robert Graves was a nineteenth-century Irish physician who first recognized this condition and consequently named it after himself. Graves' disease is caused when the body's immune system attacks the thyroid gland, especially the TSH receptors. Even after these receptors have been destroyed, the thyroid gland continues to release hormones into the bloodstream, flooding the body with excessive hormones, much like an engaged accelerator that is stuck in a car.

Graves' disease usually affects women between the ages of twenty and forty. Approximately 1 percent of the general population has Graves' disease.[4]

SIGNS AND SYMPTOMS

The most common symptoms of Graves' disease include a rapid pulse and heart palpitations. A person afflicted with this disease may even develop an arrhythmia of the heart, or atrial fibrillation, and it may cause heart failure in older patients.

Other symptoms are multiple and varied. Usually the thyroid gland is enlarged and firm. There is often a loss of muscle mass, which may cause extreme weakness.

Aside from the more common symptoms like those listed earlier in the Health Fact, another symptom is weight loss, especially loss of muscle mass. Thyroid eye disease, or *exophthalmus*, is commonly associated with Graves' disease. Those with this problem seem to have bulging, watery eyes due to eyelid retraction in which the upper eyelid is pulled back, exposing more of the white of the eyes. About half of those with Graves' disease suffer from thyroid eye disease. However, the condition usually is mild and doesn't progress once the hyperthyroidism is controlled.

A final symptom of Graves' disease is a thyroid skin disease called *pretibial myxedema*. It is much less common than thyroid eye disease and only becomes severe in about 1 percent of Graves' disease sufferers. Thyroid skin disease looks like a thickening of the skin, usually in the front of the lower leg, which becomes raised and pink.

About 10 to 15 percent of those with Graves' disease have thyroid nodules, or small lumps in the thyroid. Let's take a look.

THYROID NODULES

While they can be disturbing to think about at first, nodules of the thyroid gland are fairly common. In fact, about one in every fifteen women and one in every sixty men have a thyroid nodule—and they may not even know it![5]

A nodule is simply a small lump on the thyroid gland. It can be the size of a small pea to the size of a ping-pong ball or even larger. The good news is that the majority of thyroid nodules—in fact, over 90 percent—are benign. And even if nodules do become cancerous, they are curable about 90 percent of the time.

If you have a thyroid nodule, ask your doctor to perform thyroid function tests. Get a "free T4" and a TSH test, and also have a fine needle aspiration biopsy. ("Free T4" is the actual name of the blood test.) Some doctors perform thyroid scans as well as thyroid ultrasound studies to check a thyroid nodule, but a fine needle biopsy is a more specific procedure that may allow you to skip the thyroid scan and the ultrasound.

GOITERS

Approximately 200 million people worldwide suffer from goiters, a disturbing condition that appears as a swelling in the front of the neck.[6] A goiter is simply a swelling of the thyroid gland—a structural disorder that may be caused by Graves' or Hashimoto's disease. Another type of goiter that may occur in postmenopausal women is a multinodular goiter. Here, instead of the thyroid developing one lump, it develops multiple nodules, which are usually benign.

Causes of goiters

Goiters can be due to a number of factors: iodine insufficiency, hyperthyroidism, hypothyroidism and multinodular goiters. Most of the time, a goiter indicates that the thyroid gland is straining to produce enough hormones. However, it could also mean you are not getting enough iodine in your diet.

"Goiter Belts" was a term used to refer to areas of the country in which people often did not have adequate amounts of iodine in their diets—resulting in goiters. The Great Lakes region was once considered a goiter belt. Fortunately, goiters caused by iodine deficiency have all but been eliminated in the United States due to the development of iodized salt.

A WISE CREATOR

The psalmist said, "Bless the LORD, O my soul, and forget none of His benefits; who pardons all your iniquities, who heals all your diseases; who redeems your life from the pit, who crowns you with loving-kindness and compassion; who satisfies your years with good things, so that your youth is renewed like the eagle" (Ps. 103:2–5, NASB). This passage holds a promise that God intends to heal you of every disease—and that includes thyroid disease. He will crown you with His wonderful love and fill your years with good things.

What a wonderful promise from a wise and loving Creator. Best yet, it is not just *a* promise; it is *your* promise. Why not bow your head for a minute and thank Him for His love and healing power in your life.

A **BIBLE CURE** Prayer for You

Heavenly Father, I praise You because I am fearfully and wonderfully made. I ask that You touch my thyroid gland right now and cause it to begin to function normally. I pray that You give my doctors the wisdom to understand the root cause of this thyroid disorder and to target the most effective treatment. Please restore my body from the top of my head to the soles of my feet so that I can carry out my divine purpose in the world. In Jesus' name, amen.

A **BIBLE CURE** *Prescription*

Write a prayer concerning your current physical and emotional condition. Close it by thanking God for His healing touch.

_____

_____

_____

_____

_____

_____

_____

_____

_____

_____

_____

_____

_____

_____

_____

_____

_____

_____

_____

Chapter 11

FULL OF LIGHT—LIFESTYLE FACTORS

G LOWING HEALTH THROUGHOUT your body is a shining light. The Bible suggests that your physical well-being is directly linked to how clearly you see God's light of truth and wisdom. Luke 11:34 says, "Your eye is like a lamp that provides light for your body. When your eye is healthy, your whole body is filled with light. But when it is unhealthy, your body is filled with darkness" (NLT). In other words, seeing things in the light of God's truth shines a radiant beacon of good health and healing power throughout your body.

In God's healing light, no sickness, disease or affliction can hide. It's my prayer that your body might be full of light, with God's wisdom and truth bringing every system into perfect divine health. That is God's very best for you—body, mind and spirit.

Together let's shine the light of truth upon hidden lifestyle factors that may be at the root of your thyroid problems.

WILL THE REAL CULPRIT PLEASE STAND UP?

Diseases and their roots are part of Satan's subtle plan to defeat us— they are part of his evil arsenal, which the Bible calls "deeds of darkness." That's why disease often works in our bodies similar to the way that sin works in the soul. It hides in the darkness of our ignorance where it can do the most damage to our health. The Bible tells us we can counter darkness by exposing it to light. Ephesians 5:11, 13 says, "Take no part in the worthless deeds of evil and darkness; instead, expose them....But their evil intentions will be exposed when the light shines on them" (NLT).

In the case of thyroid disorder, there generally is one underlying culprit that is the source of the illness. Interestingly, 90 percent of all thyroid disorders can be traced to this one root problem: a malfunctioning immune system, otherwise known as an *autoimmune disorder.*[1]

Our immune system was created by God to protect us against "invaders" of our bodies—such as germs and viruses—that, if left unchecked, would cause us harm and make us sick. A strong and balanced immune system will keep us in good physical health. In the case of autoimmune disorders, the immune system itself is the cause of the illness. The immune system becomes confused and mistakes healthy organs and tissues in the body for hostile invaders, attacking them and sometimes causing serious damage. Autoimmune disorders include rheumatoid arthritis, lupus, multiple sclerosis, type 1 diabetes, ulcerative colitis, Crohn's disease, psoriasis and scleroderma. And now we know that most thyroid disease is also caused by an autoimmune disorder.

The most common cause of *hyperthyroidism* is Graves' disease; for *hypothyroidism* the most common cause is Hashimoto's thyroiditis. Both of these diseases are autoimmune disorders in which the immune system mistakes the thyroid gland for an invader and attacks it.

WHY THE CONFUSION?

There are a number of different triggers for autoimmune disorders, some of which include pregnancy, exposure to x-rays or radiation and severe emotional stress. However, one reason your immune system gets confused may be due to our contaminated environment. (See *The Bible Cure for Autoimmune Diseases* for more information.) We come into contact with thousands of chemicals every day in our food, water and air. These man-made chemicals disrupt our hormonal balance and may be the reason for a virtual onslaught of autoimmune disorders in our country—almost at epidemic proportions.

> One day while Jesus was teaching, some Pharisees and teachers of religious law were sitting nearby....And the Lord's healing power was strongly with Jesus.
>
> —LUKE 5:17, NLT

Since the beginning of the Industrial Revolution, we have poured dangerous chemicals and pollutants into our streams, soil and air. Many are nonbiodegradable, which means they take many years to break down. That's not just in the earth, but in the human body as well! One of the main jobs of our liver is to detoxify our bodies, keeping them internally cleansed from outside pollutants. But because our bodies were never intended to cope with the hefty load of chemicals they are receiving from our polluted environment, these chemicals usually become stored within our fatty tissues. From there they may begin to confuse our immune systems. Eventually our confused immune systems may begin to attack our bodies, resulting in autoimmune diseases.

TRICKING YOUR BODY

Many of the pollutants you are exposed to every day are very similar to your body's hormones, chemically speaking. So close are they, in fact, that they can trick your body into accepting them as if they were the real thing. This is where the confusion usually begins.

These pollutants come in the form of "hormone blockers," "hormone-disrupting agents" or "hormone mimickers." Some common hormone-disrupting agents include herbicides, insecticides and fungicides.

PCBs

One well-known hormone disrupter is the *polychlorinated biphenyls*—PCBs—first introduced to the environment in 1929. PCBs were used in the electronic industry as hydraulic fluid, a lubricant and a liquid seal. They were also used in consumer products to preserve rubber, to waterproof stucco and as a basic ingredient in paint, varnish and ink. Because of their proven harmful properties, PCBs were banned in 1976. However, because of their previous widespread use, they are still rampant in our environment—beyond the reach of any government recall.[2]

> O Lord, if you heal me, I will be truly healed; if you save me, I will be truly saved. My praises are for you alone!
>
> —Jeremiah 17:14, NLT

Plastic containers and wraps

Plasticizers, another less well-known hormone disrupter, come from particles of plastic wrap that "migrate" into cling-wrapped food. When meat or vegetables have been wrapped in plastic in the grocery store or slices of cheese have been individually wrapped, these foods tend to absorb the plasticizers from the wrap. When you eat this food, the plasticizers enter your body and may begin to disrupt your hormones and eventually may disrupt your immune system.

Most plastic bottles, including two-liter soda and even water bottles, contain *phthalates*, a hormone disrupter that seeps from the plastic into the soda or the water and can eventually cause health problems. It usually takes several months before the phthalates actually seep into the liquid, so it is best to buy soda or bottled water as soon after the bottling date as possible. Also, the more flexible the plastic bottle is usually indicates the more phthalates it contains. Therefore larger, thicker bottles, such as five-gallon water tanks, are safer.

Unsafe drinking water

A chemical known as *perchlorate*, which is used in rocket fuel, also has contaminated the drinking water of many different communities around the country, including Lake Mead, Nevada, and communities along the Colorado River. Perchlorate causes increased rates of hypothyroidism in newborns and can also interfere with adult thyroid function.[3]

Dental fillings

Mercury amalgams, better known as silver fillings, have been used in dentistry for over 150 years. They are actually composed of several different metals, including silver, mercury, copper and tin. The World Health Organization has estimated that the largest source of mercury in humans comes from amalgam teeth fillings—more than from all other environmental sources combined.[4] Mercury contributes to thyroid disease by binding to the thyroid gland and disrupting its function. For more information on this topic, refer to my book *What You Don't Know May Be Killing You.*

ARE YOU A POOR CONVERTER?

I mentioned earlier that most of the thyroid hormone in your body—about 80 percent—is called T4. T4 is important; however, another thyroid hormone is even more important. T3 is the active form of thyroid hormone (which is the hormone that actually does most of the work) and is several times stronger than T4. So, in order for your cells to get the hormone (T3) that it needs, it must change or convert the T4 to T3.

This chemical change takes place mainly in the liver and to a less extent in the kidneys and muscles.

> Jesus traveled throughout the region of Galilee...[and] healed every kind of disease and illness.
> —MATTHEW 4:23, NLT

Many individuals whose thyroid test results are normal but who still have symptoms of hypothyroidism are simply *poor converters* of T4 to the T3 hormone. This can result from too many toxins in the liver, free-radical damage or impaired enzyme function. Below are some other lifestyle factors that can make you a poor converter or that may interfere with thyroid function.

Stress

Excessive stress can lead to adrenal fatigue, which, in turn, may lead to problems converting T4 to T3. This is especially true after your body has been through a protracted illness, a chronic injury from an accident, the stress of surgery or emotional stress. (For more information on stress, refer to *The Bible Cure for Stress.*)

Aging

As you get older, it becomes increasingly difficult for your body to keep converting T4 to T3 efficiently.

Cigarette smoking

Chronic cigarette smoking causes problems with thyroid hormone conversion.

Excessive fluoride

Fluoride has been added to most toothpaste and public drinking water to prevent cavities and tooth decay. However, too much fluoride can result in a decrease in thyroid function. Interestingly, fluoride was once used as a medication to *slow down* an overactive thyroid!

Excessive chlorine

Chlorine is added to water—including our drinking water—to kill microorganisms. However, similar to the effect of excessive fluoride, chlorine can interfere with proper thyroid hormone conversion, and excessive intake may result in hypothyroidism.

Certain medications

Certain medications can either trigger or aggravate hypothyroidism. For example, lithium blocks the uptake of iodine, which is necessary for thyroid function, and inhibits the production and release of the thyroid hormone. Amiodarone is a medication prescribed for certain cardiac arrhythmias, but it is linked to hypothyroidism in approximately 10 percent of patients who take it.

Other medications can interfere with thyroid function, such as the antifungal drug Nizoral; antibiotics such as Bactrim and Septra; and certain diabetic drugs such as Orinase and Diabinese. Other medications, including estrogen, birth control pills, anabolic steroids and prednisone, can all affect thyroid function. Even beta blockers used to treat hypertension (such as Inderal and Tenormin) can affect thyroid function. You should always ask your physician or consult with a *Physician's Desk Reference* to determine if your medication is affecting your thyroid function.

Any of the factors named above, including being around too many toxins, may be the reason you are experiencing symptoms of low thyroid. I strongly suggest that you take immediate measures to minimize or eliminate these lifestyle factors. (For more information on this topic, read my book *Toxic Relief.*)

Stop smoking, and if you are taking synthetic hormones, discuss natural alternatives with your health provider. Minimize stress, and if you've had major surgery or experienced an injury, be sure to allow your body time to recover completely. If you are taking birth control pills and experiencing many symptoms of thyroid disease, consider asking your doctor about other methods.

OTHER FACTORS MAY PLACE YOU AT RISK

Even if you do not smoke, have no amalgam fillings, don't take synthetic hormones and live in a relatively pollution-free environment, other factors still may be placing you at greater risk for thyroid disease.

Listed below are high-risk factors for developing hypothyroidism.

Family history

If you have a close family member—a parent, sibling, grandparent, aunt or uncle—with a thyroid disorder, your risk is higher.

Pregnancy

If you are pregnant, know that it is fairly common for women to develop postpartum hypothyroidism just after pregnancy. However, don't be alarmed. Most women's thyroid function returns to normal when the hormones associated with pregnancy and lactation also return to normal. However, hypothyroidism will continue in some women, and steps must be taken to restore thyroid function in these patients.

> He sent out his word and healed them, snatching them from the door of death.
> —PSALM 107:20, NLT

Exposure to radiation

Exposure to radiation, especially from receiving radioactive iodine, can increase your risk of developing hypothyroidism. Before 1970, radiation and x-ray treatments were used to treat diseases from acne to tonsillitis—even colds and adenoid problems. Today these treatments are being linked to thyroid nodules, hypothyroidism and even thyroid cancer.

Radioactive iodine has been a common treatment for Graves' disease, which in many cases leads to hypothyroidism. Thyroid surgery, such as for thyroid cancer or for large goiters, may also lead to hypothyroidism.

In Hosea 4:6, God tells us, "My people are destroyed for lack of knowledge" (NASB). But it doesn't have to be this way! God has given us the knowledge that we need to combat thyroid disorders. Even though we live in a toxic earth, we don't have to succumb to autoimmune disorders. We can start cleansing our bodies and decreasing our stress by taking steps to change our lifestyle habits. (Refer to my books *Toxic Relief, What You Don't Know May Be Killing You* and *The Bible Cure for Autoimmune Diseases* for information on these topics.)

LIVE IN THE LIGHT

As you continue to read through this Bible Cure book, the Lord is lighting a path of understanding for you so that no hidden problem can rob you of your health. The psalmist wrote, "You light a lamp for me. The LORD, My God, lights up my darkness" (Ps. 18:28, NLT). Allow Him, and He will light a pathway into His own healing, restoring, cleansing presence that you've never before imagined was possible. He invites you to walk in the light of His wonderful love.

> Have compassion on me, LORD, for I am weak.
>
> —PSALM 6:2, NLT

If you long to know Him better, if you seek His healing touch, ask Him now, "Lord, let me live in the light of Your truth." If you think you may have a thyroid condition that is due to an underlying autoimmune disorder, pray the following prayer with me right now.

A **BIBLE CURE** *Prayer for You*

Heavenly Father, You created my body to function in perfect harmony, and my immune system was intended to protect me from any outside invaders that would cause me harm. God, it is not Your will that my immune system is confused and attacking my thyroid gland, and that it is an unhealthy invader. I thank You for restoring order and peace within my body right now and that all of my bodily systems line up with Your Word. In Jesus' name, amen.

A **BIBLE CURE** *Prescription*

Take an inventory of the disruptive agents to which you are exposed in your daily lifestyle.

❏ What sources of plastic pollution do you encounter daily?

❏ Is your mouth filled with silver (mercury) fillings?

❏ What other disruptive agents and medications do you feel may be affecting your health?

❏ Are you willing to trust God to help you change your lifestyle and lessen your health risk from environmental contaminants?

Chapter 12

BRIGHTER AND BRIGHTER—
SUPPLEMENTS

M ANY BELIEVE THAT God's teachings are for our mind and spirit only. Yet, God created our entire being—body, mind and spirit. If we allow Him, He will teach us wisdom to light a pathway of healing and understanding. The Bible says, "For their command is a lamp and their instruction a light" (Prov. 6:23, NLT).

God is determined to stop your enemies of sickness and disease from keeping you from His perfect plan for your life. Psalm 30:1–2 says, "You refused to let my enemies triumph over me. O LORD my God, I cried out to you for help, and you restored my health" (NLT).

No matter how dark your circumstances or physical symptoms may seem at the moment, when you look to God for help they get brighter and brighter. "The way of the righteous is like the first gleam of dawn, which shines ever brighter until the full light of day" (Prov. 4:18, NLT).

So, be encouraged, and get ready to start feeling much better, for there is much you can do to turn your situation completely around. You have already seen how lifestyle factors can make a great difference in how your thyroid functions. Let's shine the light a little brighter by taking a look at some natural substances God has placed in His great creation that can help you gain victory.

> Dear friend, I hope all is well with you and that you are as healthy in body as you are strong in spirit.
>
> —3 JOHN 2, NLT

NECESSARY NUTRIENTS FOR A HEALTHY THYROID

Iodine

Iodine, from seawater, is a natural substance found in abundance throughout the earth. As we've seen, getting too little or too much iodine can dramatically impact thyroid health. Too much can lead to hyperthyroidism and can actually trigger the autoimmune response, and too little can lead to goiters and other thyroid problems. Low iodine levels are actually a leading cause of thyroid dysfunction in the world at large, although it is not as great a factor in developed countries such the U.S. and European countries where table salt is iodized.

Yet, many Americans who have banned all salt from their diets for health reasons are starting to experience problems. More and more bakeries and restaurants also feature low-salt or no-salt selections. A study in the *Journal of Clinical Endocrinology and Metabolism* in October of 1998 showed that the iodine levels measured in urine excretion had fallen by half compared to tests of earlier studies done for people living in the U.S. It cited that 12 percent of Americans had low iodine concentrations in their urine compared to 1994, when less than 1 percent of the population had low levels of iodine.[1]

The American Heart Association recommends that we get a teaspoon of salt every day (6 grams, which contains approximately 400 mcg of iodine).[2]

Since nature's primary source of iodine is seawater, the closer you live to the sea the better off you are, at least in respect to getting enough iodine in your body. If you live in the central plains or near the Great Lakes, then your body is dependent upon the iodine you receive in your table salt and food that comes from the sea.

> They begged him [Jesus] to let the sick touch at least the fring of his robe, and all who touched him were healed.
> —MARK 6:56, NLT

If you are on a low-salt diet and rarely eat ocean fish and seafood, onions or dairy products, I recommend taking a daily multivitamin/multimineral supplement that contains 150 mcg of iodine. Use iodized salt or, even better, use sea salt or Celtic salt. The RDA for adults is 150 mcg a day, and, fortunately, the usual daily intake in the U.S. is about 150 to 550 mcg per day.

Caution: Balance is very important where iodine is involved, for we've seen that it can be a double-edged sword. Too much or too little iodine can lead to thyroid problems. Therefore, do not take large doses of kelp or other supplements high in iodine since they may trigger hyperthyroidism.

Tyrosine

The thyroid gland actually needs two different nutrients from the diet: the first is iodine, and the second is *tyrosine*. Tyrosine is an amino acid that the body forms from the metabolism of the essential amino acid *phenylalanine*. In fact, the body makes most of the tyrosine it needs from phenylalanine, so tyrosine is not considered an essential amino acid to add to the diet, although it is helpful to do so.

Foods that are high in tyrosine include chicken, fish, soybeans, bananas, dairy foods, almonds and lima beans. Be sure to include plenty of these items in your regular diet in order to get enough tyrosine.

Let's take a look at some supplements that will give good results.

Super Supplements

If you have a thyroid disorder, or a borderline thyroid disorder, supplements can help bring your body back into the right balance. Here are some supplements you may take.

A good multivitamin/multimineral

Your multivitamin should contain vitamin A, vitamin B_2, B_6, B_{12}, vitamin C and zinc. Moderate amounts of these substances are essential for making thyroid hormone. Zinc is essential, but it must also be balanced with copper in a 10:1 ratio. It's unwise to economize when it comes to vitamins, since quality varies widely among brands. The best brands generally will yield the best results. Divine Health Multivitamins is a high-quality brand. You can order it from my Web site at www.drcolbert.com.

Selenium

Selenium, an important antioxidant, is one of the most important nutrients your body uses to convert thyroid hormone to meet your body's needs. Interestingly, Brazil nuts contain a whopping 840 mcg of selenium per ounce—twelve times as much as you need each day.

The RDA for selenium is 70 mcg, so check your label as dosages can vary widely from brand to brand.

Dosage: Take a multivitamin that contains at least 100 mcg of selenium, or take a selenium supplement. You may choose to simply eat a Brazil nut a day.

Moducare and Natur-Leaf

Moducare and Natur-Leaf are blends of plant sterols and sterolins that work to restore, strengthen and balance your body's immune system. Plant sterols and sterolins are natural substances found in all fruits, vegetables, nuts and seeds.

Because they help to balance the immune system, Moducare or Natur-Leaf may prove effective in helping treat both Hashimoto's thyroiditis, the leading cause of hypothyroidism, and Graves' disease, the leading cause of hyperthyroidism.

> O LORD my God, I cried to you for help, and you restored my health.
>
> —PSALM 30:2, NLT

Plant sterols and sterolins generally also have an anti-inflammatory effect. They also may be able to modulate the autoimmune response. I recommend plant sterols and sterolins especially for patients with Graves' disease.

Moducare, which can be found at most health food stores, is one of the most popular of the plant sterol treatments. Natur-Leaf may be ordered by calling 1-888-532-7845.

Dosage for Moducare: Adults can take one capsule three times daily, or two capsules upon rising and one at bedtime. This dose may need to be increased to two to three capsules three times per day, taken one hour before meals. The dose for Natur-Lear is generally one capsule two times a day one hour before meals, but it may need to be increased to two capsules two times a day. Since Moducare and Natur-Leaf are similar products, I recommend that you take one or the other.

A MARVELOUS SYMPHONY

Do you remember the old children's song "Dry Bones"? The song went on and on about each part of the body being connected to the other parts of the body.

The incredible intricacy and complexity of the human body can never be fully expressed in a children's song. That's because your body's complex systems work together like a marvelous symphony orchestrated to perfection, with each part vitally connected to the others, working together to keep you healthy and happy.

The endocrine system, which is made up of the various glands in your body, is a vital part of that grand symphony. Each gland is interconnected and communicates with all of the other glands. The hypothalamus, pituitary gland, thyroid gland, adrenal glands and reproductive glands all work closely together. When there is an imbalance in one gland, such as the adrenal glands or the reproductive glands, it can, in turn, put a strain on the functioning of the thyroid gland.

STRESSED OUT ADRENALS?

Your adrenal glands produce many different hormones, including cortisol, DHEA, progesterone, pregnenolone, testosterone and estrogen. When you are under a lot of stress for a prolonged period of time, these vitally important glands can begin producing excessive cortisol. Excessive cortisol production may eventually lead to adrenal fatigue and possibly adrenal exhaustion accompanied by low cortisol production. Both of these states—excessive cortisol production and low cortisol production—can make you a poor converter of T4 to T3. Remember, T3 is the active form of thyroid hormone and is several times stronger than T4.

DSF

During extended times of stress, you can help your body to balance its production of cortisol by supplementing with DSF. This de-stress formula is carefully blended to help restore the body's adrenal function. You can purchase this excellent supplement from Nutri-West by calling 1-800-451-5620.

Dosage: Take at least one chewable tablet twice a day at breakfast and lunch.

DHEA

DHEA is a hormone made naturally by your adrenal glands. Many call it the "youth" hormone because low levels are linked to aging. When your adrenals are exhausted, often your supply of DHEA is low, which causes hormonal regulation in your entire body to suffer. When your cortisol levels are high, DHEA levels are usually low. You can replenish this vital hormone by taking it in supplement form.

Dosage: Take a small amount of DHEA under the tongue once a day (women 5 mg a day; men, 10 mg a day).

For more information on the adrenal glands, please refer to *The Bible Cure for Stress.* To order DHEA, visit our Web site at www.drcolbert.com.

A **BIBLE CURE** Health Tip

Screen Your Own Adrenals

You can screen yourself to find out if your adrenal glands are functioning optimally. Here's how.

The Blood Pressure Test

Take your own blood pressure while lying down after you've been at rest for a moderate length of time. Record your reading in the space below.

_____

Stand up and immediately take your blood pressure again. Write it in the space below.

_____

Evaluation: (check one)
- ❏ My blood pressure stayed the same.
- ❏ My blood pressure rose.
- ❏ My blood pressure dropped.

If your blood pressure went up or stayed the same, your adrenals are probably in fairly good shape. However, if your blood pressure dropped after you stood up, there is a good chance you are suffering from adrenal fatigue.[3]

If you are not equipped to accurately read your own blood pressure, try this test instead. You will need the help of a close friend.

The Pupil Dilation Test: Rogoff's Sign

In a dark room, have a close friend shine a flashlight directly into your eye for approximately thirty seconds. He or she will be evaluating the size of your pupil. Your pupil will need to be watched very closely.

Normal pupil: If your pupil is normal it will constrict in the light and remain small.

Abnormal pupil: If your pupil wavers, dilates or does not constrict, it is abnormal. Any of these abnormal reactions suggest your body is experiencing adrenal fatigue.

CHECK IT OUT

I strongly suggest that you have all of your hormone levels checked and that you begin supplementing any hormones you are lacking. Both those with hypothyroidism and hyperthyroidism generally have low adrenal reserves and would benefit greatly from DHEA and DSF.

Natural testosterone or progesterone

One final note: Because of the close association between the various glands—including the reproductive glands—I have found that many people with thyroid disorders have low levels of sex hormones.

If you have a thyroid disorder, you may need to have your sex hormones checked. Women may need phytoestrogens and a natural progesterone cream, along with small amounts of natural testosterone cream. Salivary hormone testing of adrenal hormones and sex hormones is a simple test to screen for imbalances of these hormones.

TAKE WARNING

You may be especially health conscious and currently take several supplements in order to strengthen your body. But if you have a thyroid disorder, you may need to reexamine what you're taking. Some supplements may actually aggravate your condition.

Lipoic acid

Lipoic acid is a powerful antioxidant used by many physicians to treat diabetes, hepatitis and psoriasis. However, lipoic acid may make you a poor converter, decreasing your ability to convert T4 to T3. That's the reason that some people who take lipoic acid begin exhibiting many of the symptoms of hypothyroidism.

If you have begun to take lipoic acid and have developed several symptoms of a low thyroid, you may need to either lower your dose or stop taking it altogether.

Kelp and bladderwrack

These herbs are known for having many health benefits, but they also contain lots of iodine. And as you've seen, too much iodine can increase your risk for developing hyperthyroidism. That's especially true if you are getting plenty of iodine in your table salt.

If you have symptoms of thyroid disorder and are taking either of these herbs, I encourage you to find other supplements containing less iodine.

TREATING HYPOTHYROIDISM
Synthetic (man-made) preparations

If you have hypothyroidism, no supplement or herb can substitute for what you really need, which is thyroid hormone. Your physician will probably start you on T4, which is supplied by the major synthetic brands of T4 thyroid hormones (Synthroid, Levothroid, Levoxyl and Unithroid). Some patients, for whatever reason, don't respond as well to generic synthetic T4 hormone preparations, and so I recommend that you take the major brands mentioned above.

> Don't be afraid, for I am with you. Don't be discouraged, for I am your God. I will strengthen you and help you. I will hold you up with my victorious right hand.
>
> —ISAIAH 41:10, NLT

Synthetic T4 thyroid hormones are the standard treatment of choice for most doctors. Very rarely will a medical doctor stray from prescribing one of the four preparations listed above, or a generic version of them. Synthroid remains the top-selling thyroid hormone in the United States—its generic substitute is called *levothyroxine.*

As you have learned, many patients are unable to successfully convert the T4 hormone to T3, yet their thyroid tests are normal. For these patients, the synthetic T3 hormone called *liothyronine* may be effective. Its product name is *Cytomel.* A small amount of Cytomel in a sustained-released preparation will often relieve the symptoms of hypothyroidism in these individuals. These sustained released preparations of thyroid hormone can only be obtained from a compounding pharmacy such as Pharmacy Specialists. Your physician can contact them at 1-407-260-7002.

Most physicians, however, only prescribe the T4 hormone such as Synthroid. I believe that in the future, more doctors will begin to provide an appropriate mixture of T4 and T3, which is more similar to the actual hormone secretion of the thyroid gland.

A MORE NATURAL PATH

Perhaps you've determined that you prefer to treat your hypothyroidism condition with more natural methods. Staying as close to nature as possible is often best. Nevertheless, you may imagine that only those with borderline thyroid disease have that option. But you're wrong. Natural medications exist even for those with long-term hypothyroidism. Let's take a look at some more natural options.

Natural thyroid hormone preparations, including Armour Thyroid, Biotech Thyroid, Westhroid and Naturethroid, are medications produced from the desiccated thyroid glands of pigs. They contain both T4 and T3 hormones. Each of these natural thyroid products is essentially the same—they just have different fillers. One important note: If you have allergies to corn, take the Biotech or Naturethroid products, which have no corn fillers.

> Your wouds will quickly heal. Your godliness will lead you forward, and the glory of the LORD will protect you from behind.
> —ISAIAH 58:8, NLT

With my own patients, I generally prescribe a natural thyroid hormone such as those listed above.

Again, many individuals with hypothyroidism take some form of synthetic T4, usually Synthroid, but may not be getting all the T3 they need, since many are poor converters of T4 to T3. This is the reason why they may continue to exhibit symptoms of hypothyroidism. By switching to a natural thyroid hormone or simply by adding a small amount of sustained-release T3, most symptoms of hypothyroidism can be eliminated.

A **BIBLE CURE** Health Tip

Tips for Taking Thyroid Hormone Supplements

❏ Take thyroid hormone mediations about the same time each day.

❏ Don't take thyroid medication with other medications.

❏ It is critically important to take the thyroid hormone on an empty stomach with water so that it can be absorbed efficiently.

❏ Do not take thyroid hormones with iron supplements—wait at least two to three hours after taking the thyroid hormone before taking an iron supplement.

❏ Wait at least three to four hours after taking a thyroid supplement before taking any calcium. This includes milk and even orange juice, since most orange juice has been fortified with calcium.

❏ Take multivitamins, which generally contain both iron and calcium, at least three hours after taking the thyroid hormone.

❏ Do not take antacids, such as Maalox or Mylanta, with the thyroid hormone. Wait at least two to three hours after taking a thyroid hormone before taking these medications.

GAINING AGAINST GRAVES'

The standard medical treatment for Graves' disease, which is hyperthyroidism, has benefits and also a downside. Let's take a look.

Radioactive iodine

The most common treatment for Graves' disease is radioactive iodine 131 (RAI). This treatment actually destroys cells in the thyroid gland so that it becomes unable to produce thyroid hormone. Unfortunately, many patients who undergo this treatment go to the other extreme and develop hypothyroidism.

Antithyroid medication

For my patients with Graves' disease, I prefer to prescribe antithyroid medication, particularly methimazole or Tapazole. This medication blocks the production of thyroid hormone without destroying the cells of the thyroid gland itself.

ARMED WITH UNDERSTANDING

The next time you see your doctor, you will go armed with a greater understanding about your thyroid condition. Realize too that, with the power of the knowledge you have gained in this book, you now have more than one choice of medication. Most doctors will simply prescribe Synthroid (synthetic T4), but you've gained the option of finding a physician who can prescribe a natural thyroid medication, such as Armour Thyroid, Naturethroid or Biotech Thyroid. Even if you cannot find such a doctor, your own doctor might be willing to add T3 hormone to your regimen.

> He comforts us in all our troubles so that we can comfort others. When they are troubled, we will be able to give them the same comfort God has given us.
>
> —2 CORINTHIANS 1:4, NLT

A GREAT PHYSICIAN

Wisdom and knowledge alone are not enough in themselves. As you seek healing for your condition, always seek the Healer first. All healing comes from Him.

Often His healing power comes into your life as a rising light that shines with greater and greater power as it flows into you and through you to everyone you meet. The Bible says, "The Sun of Righteousness will rise with healing in his wings" (Mal. 4:2, NLT). I believe this brightness of His rising is already beginning to shine upon your life.

Fortunately, we have the Great Physician on our side, the One who possesses all the keys to knowledge and wisdom and who loves us with an everlasting love. Turn to Him and begin to seek His wisdom and healing power.

A BIBLE CURE Prayer for You

Dear heavenly Father, I know that You are the Creator of the universe and the Creator of my body. I thank You that You understand the mysterious intricacies that make up the systems of my body and that it is Your will that they all function together in perfect harmony. Lord, I place my thyroid gland and all of its functions into Your capable hands. You are the Healer, the Great Physician, and I trust You with my condition. Teach me the things that I need to do, the areas I may need to change, in order to walk in Your divine health. And give me the grace and the discipline I need to follow through. In Jesus' name, amen.

A **BIBLE CURE** *Prescription*

List the supplements you are planning to speak with your physician about taking.

_____

_____

_____

What sources of iodine are you getting in your diet?

_____

_____

_____

Based upon the information you read in this chapter, should you make any changes to your iodine intake? If so, what are they?

_____

_____

_____

What good multivitamin/multimineral supplement are you taking at present?

_____

_____

_____

What sources of selenium are you presently getting in your diet?

_____

_____

_____

Do you believe you may be a poor converter of T4 to T3? Why?

_____

_____

_____

Chapter 13

A LIGHTED TEMPLE—NUTRITION

WALKING IN THE light of God's wisdom will actually change your physical appearance. The Bible says, "How wonderful to be wise, to analyze and interpret things. Wisdom lights up a person's face, softening its hardness" (Eccles. 8:1, NLT).

In fact, your entire being can shine in the light of God's truth. The Book of Daniel says, "Those who are wise will shine like the brightness of the firmament, and those who turn many to righteousness like the stars forever and ever" (Dan. 12:3, NKJV).

Daniel was a wise young man who had a spirit of excellence. Interestingly, one of the ways he displayed excellence that pleased God greatly was through his dietary choices. For when the banquets of kings were placed before him, menus that were doubtless filled with fatty meats, sugary sweets and the most refined breads and cakes available in the kingdom, Daniel refused to indulge. Even at the risk of punishment, he chose to eat only vegetables. Why? He wisely understood that his food choices made a great difference in both the natural and spiritual realms. This excellent young man realized his body was a temple of the Holy Spirit, and he refused to eat anything that might defile it.

> Don't be impressed with your own wisdom. Instead, fear the LORD and turn away from evil. Then you will have healing for your body and strength for your bones.
> —PROVERBS 3:7–8, NLT

AMERICA'S RICH MAN'S DIET

Proverbs 23:1–3 says, "When dining with a ruler, pay attention to what is put before you. If you are a big eater, put a knife to your throat, and don't desire all the delicacies, for he might be trying to trick you" (NLT). Here the Bible warns us against the "deception" of eating what is pleasing to our palates but may not nourish and strengthen our bodies. In fact, much of the rich, sugary, refined foods historically eaten by the rich were genuinely bad for the body. The simpler whole-grain breads, fish and vegetables of peasants who lived closer to the natural earth were far healthier.

Amazingly, America's "rich man's diet" of excessive sweets and refined, processed foods and fatty meats has created an epidemic of sickness. It is estimated that 75 percent of all deaths each year are related to inadequate nutrition.[1] It's no wonder that God gave such a strong warning against the "deceptive food" of refined, processed and sugary items that taste good but do not adequately nourish the body.

Your body is the temple of God. First Corinthians 6:19 says, "Don't you realize that your body is the temple of the Holy Spirit, who lives in you and was given to you by God? You do not belong to yourself" (NLT). What you put into your temple will determine a great deal about your health—both physically and spiritually. Daniel refused to defile his temple. What about you?

If you have thyroid disease or its symptoms, you may need to reject certain dietary choices in order to protect and heal your body. You have an excellent spirit just like Daniel, and with God's help you can begin implementing this Bible cure step of making good nutritional choices. As God shines His wonderful Spirit upon you, your temple will be increasingly filled with His glorious light.

Let's turn now and explore this vital Bible cure step.

YOU ARE WHAT YOU EAT

An old expression says, "You are what you eat." In other words, eating good, healthy foods will give your body strong, powerful nutrients with which to build and repair itself. Providing your body with inferior nutrition can make it weak and easily susceptible to infirmity and disease.

Begin this Bible cure step by determining to rid your diet of selections that weaken your immune system and undermine your overall balance of health.

Reject

Reject all highly processed foods, refined grains, starches and sugars.

Prefer

Eat plenty of fresh vegetables, fresh fruits and unrefined, complex carbohydrates. Here's a good rule of thumb: The closer to the garden you eat, the better. The farther away from the garden—in terms of processing and refining—the worse off your food selections will be.

GO ORGANIC

Organic foods are becoming increasingly popular and easier to find. Many food chains now carry organic varieties of just about everything. The prices for organic foods are going down, too. Although organics may still cost a little more, the health benefits are well worth it. Here's why.

Fruits and vegetables

Organic fruits and vegetables will decrease your exposure to hormone-disruptive substances. These include the pesticides, synthetic hormones and other toxins we discussed in chapter 10. Therefore, as often as you can, choose organically grown vegetables and fruits. When you cannot, be aggressive in carefully washing your fruits and vegetables with warm water and a mild soap, or try using one of the popular vegetable cleansing products available at health food stores. Be sure to rinse well after washing.

Dairy products

Choose organic milk, eggs and dairy products. Non-organic varieties may contain hormones and antibiotics, both of which can dramatically impact your thyroid function. Also choose low-fat or nonfat dairy products.

Meats

Free-range meats are not fed hormones and other drugs to fatten them up. If you can afford it, choose these whenever possible. When purchasing non-free-range meats, select the leanest cuts and carefully trim off the fat and skin. Hormone-disrupting chemicals are primarily concentrated in the fat of the animal, so significantly reducing the amount of animal fat in your diet will make a big difference.

DANGER: NUTRASWEET CAN HARM YOU!

Do you drink iced tea throughout the day and add that little blue packet of sweetener? Or do you enjoy a diet soda in the afternoons? If so, the aspartame in these products could be affecting your thyroid.

Researchers are discovering that aspartame can have a dramatic negative impact on the thyroid.[2] If you have hypothyroidism, Graves' disease or Hashimoto's thyroiditis, or if you have symptoms indicating you may be developing either of these thyroid diseases, I strongly encourage you avoid using all products that contain aspartame, or NutraSweet.

OPPOSITE ENDS OF THE SPECTRUM

Because *hypothyroidism* (too little thyroid hormone) and *hyperthyroidism* (too much thyroid hormone) are opposite ends of the delicate thyroid hormone balance, those with either of these conditions will at times receive vastly different advice. Consider these thyroid disorders as book ends.

Check out the specific dietary advice concerning your particular situation very carefully. Don't be surprised to discover that you may need to do exactly the opposite of what someone at the other end of the balance scale needs to do.

SOY PRODUCTS AND YOUR THYROID

Normally I encourage my patients to eat soy products, as long as they are not allergic to them. However, eating a lot of soy products is unwise if you are struggling to overcome an underactive thyroid, or *hypothyroidism*. Soy products suppress thyroid function.

Soy products—including soybeans, soy milk and soy

protein—contain isoflavins. Isoflavins, such as *genistein*, block iodine and tyrosine, preventing them from producing the thyroid hormone. In addition, check to determine whether other supplements you are taking contain genistein or other isoflavins. If so, decrease or avoid these products that tend to suppress thyroid function further.

For those with an underactive thyroid, soy products can promote the formation of goiters as well as trigger autoimmune thyroid disease.

Now, if you have *hyperthyroidism*, or an overactive thyroid, soy products will usually prove beneficial to you, since your body is producing too much thyroid hormone and soy products tend to slow that process down.

Don't Eat These With Hypothyroidism

Certain foods are called *goitrogens* because eating them in excessive amounts can lead to the formation of goiters and hypothyroidism (an underactive thyroid). This is caused by cyanide derivatives contained in the plants. Because cooking them thoroughly usually inactivates the goitrogens, if you have low thyroid function, limit the amount of foods you consume raw; instead, steam or cook them.

Goitrogen foods primarily consist of raw vegetables, especially cruciferous ones. These include:

- Broccoli
- Cabbage
- Cauliflower
- Brussels sprouts
- Kale
- Turnip and mustard greens

Besides these vegetables, other goitrogens include:

- Sweet corn
- Millet
- Pine nuts
- Peanuts
- Almonds
- Walnuts

When these foods make up a major part of your diet, especially if eaten raw, they can create a risk factor for hypothyroidism. However, I'm not suggesting that you cut out these foods completely from your diet. Merely limit them, and steam or cook cruciferous vegetables before eating them.

Do Eat These With Hyperthyroidism

Conversely, if you have *hyperthyroidism*, certain foods that those with *hypothyroidism* must limit are actually good for you. While these foods are not good for patients who have an underactive thyroid gland, they have beneficial effects for an overactive thyroid. They can slow down a hyperactive thyroid, much like pressing on the brakes of a car. You may eat plenty of the following:

- Broccoli
- Cauliflower
- Cabbage
- Brussels sprouts
- Sweet corn
- Millet
- Peanuts
- Almonds
- Walnuts

Don't Eat These With Hyperthyroidism

Because excessive iodine intake helps promote hyperthyroidism, too much of it in your diet can intensify symptoms of hyperthyroidism when you are battling Graves' disease. Therefore, if your thyroid is overactive, limit these selections:

- Ocean fish
- Shellfish
- Dairy products
- Kelp and other forms of seaweed
- Onions

All of these selections are loaded with iodine. In addition, many bakeries add extra salt and iodine to dough to make it easier to work with. In fact, a slice of bread typically contains about 150 mcg of iodine. This is another powerful reason to limit your intake of processed foods.

Fatten Up

Another symptom of Graves' disease (an overactive thyroid) is weight loss, especially muscle mass. If you are battling hyperthyroidism, you are probably prone to losing too much muscle weight. Therefore, you need to eat a diet high in protein to counteract the muscle loss you are experiencing. I also recommend 100 mcg a day of coenzyme Q_{10} to protect the heart, which is a muscle.

Consume even more calories than usual—especially unrefined, complex carbohydrates, proteins and "good" fats. Eat often, every three to four hours, to prevent weight loss.

THE WONDER OF WATER

To combat any thyroid condition, it is extremely important to drink adequate amounts of water—at least two quarts day.

Also, stop drinking tap water; drink filtered water instead. Reverse-osmosis-filtered water is some of the cleanest water you can drink, and it generally doesn't contain hormone-disrupting chemicals, fluoride, chlorine or other chemicals, which can affect the thyroid.

If you decide to drink bottled water, make sure that you know the date that the water was bottled, and drink it as close to that date as possible—at least within a month or two—in order to decrease your exposure to plasticizers or phthalates.

A **BIBLE CURE** Health Tip

How Much Water Do I Need?

Here's a good way to find out how much water you really need to drink every day.

❏ Write down your weight in pounds   _____
❏ Divide that number by 2   _____
❏ Remainder =   _____

The remainder is the number of ounces of water you need to drink daily.

BE A DOER

The Bible encourages us, "Be ye doers of the word, and not hearers only" (James 1:22, KJV). This is good advice, even as it applies to practical nutritional wisdom for good health. By learning about and implementing these simple health strategies, you are now armed with the knowledge you need to combat your thyroid disorder. Knowledge is power, and when put into use, it becomes wisdom for prevention and healing for yourself and others.

A **BIBLE CURE** *Prayer for You*

Lord Jesus, thank You so much for the knowledge and wisdom You have provided in this book. I ask You for Your help and guidance as I begin to implement these strategies in my life. Continue to further the healing that You have begun in my body as I learn to walk in Your ways. Thank You for Your healing power that is always available to me. As I go forth in health and wholeness, I will share Your love and mercy with others and begin to follow the plan that You have designed for my life. In Jesus' name I pray all of these things, amen.

A **BIBLE CURE** Prescription

Write your particular thyroid condition in the space below.

_____

_____

What foods will you eat to help with your healing?

_____

_____

What foods will you reject?

_____

_____

How much water do you drink per day?

_____

_____

How much should you be drinking according to the Health Tip in this chapter?

_____

_____

Write out a strategy to help you drink more water every day.

_____

_____

Record your commitment to God to be a doer and not a hearer only.

_____

_____

Chapter 14

ARISE, SHINE—FAITH

WHEN YOUR BODY is bright with a radiant glow of vibrant health, your light will shine to others all around you. The Bible says, "Then Jesus asked them, 'Would anyone light a lamp and then put it under a basket or under a bed? Of course not! A lamp is placed on a stand, where its light will shine'" (Mark 4:21, NLT).

This book would be incomplete without the final Bible cure step: faith. In order to walk in the radiant glow of health that God intends for you, you must step out in faith and boldly receive His very best.

WHAT IS FAITH?

Faith is not a dove or a cloud. It's not a gift that some have and others lack. It's not an eerie force, and it's not the "luck of the draw" or what happens to those who win the lottery.

Faith is choosing to believe God, no matter what anyone else says, no matter what your eyes see or your ears hear. Faith determines to choose to believe that God is your healer, that He loves you and that He desires to see you well.

Right now you have all the faith you need to experience a total healing in your body. The Bible says all it takes is a little, tiny kernel of faith, no bigger than a mustard seed.

Faith simply takes God at His Word. That's why faith is simple enough for a child to grasp.

RISE AND SHINE

The Book of Isaiah commands, "Arise, shine; for your light has come, and the glory of the LORD has risen upon you" (Isa. 60:1, NASB). Faith always demands action. You must be the one who determines to arise.

When you do so, you can be sure that you will shine because the glorious light of God's presence will rise upon your life.

Why not choose to rise up in faith and claim God's promises this very moment? If bold, unwavering faith is your choice right now, then step out on God's promise by bowing your head and praying this prayer. Get ready to let your light shine brightly!

A **BIBLE CURE** Prayer for You

Lord Jesus, You are the amazing Healer. You hold the keys to all power, wisdom and understanding—the very earth itself was created by Your will and Your hand. But I know that You are also my Savior—that You bore the stripes on Your back so that my healing could take place. Lord, I trust You with my condition. I believe that You have the power to heal me, and not only that, You want to heal me! I place myself in Your hands and ask that Your healing power would flow in me and through me. Let the healing of my condition take place and be a witness and a testimony to Your power and love. I declare today that I choose faith. I receive Your healing power right now. In Jesus' name, amen.

A **Bible Cure** *Prescription*

Faith Builder

He was pierced through for our transgressions, He was crushed for our iniquities; the chastening for our well-being fell upon Him, and by His scourging we are healed.

—Isaiah 53:5, nas

Read this dynamic scripture aloud several times. It has great power! Insert your own name into it.

He was pierced through for _____ transgressions, He was crushed for _____ iniquities; the chastening of _____ well-being fell upon Him, and by His scourging _____ is healed!

Now write a prayer thanking God for your healing.

_____

_____

_____

_____

_____

_____

_____

_____

_____

_____

_____

_____

_____

_____

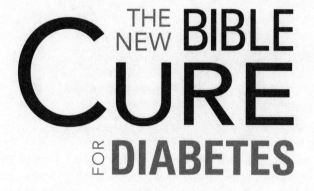

THE NEW BIBLE
CURE
FOR DIABETES

Chapter 15

A NEW BIBLE CURE WITH NEW
HOPE FOR DIABETES

G OD'S DESIRE IS for you to feel better and to live longer, and He will help you reach that goal! By picking up this revised and expanded Bible Cure book, you have taken an exciting first step toward renewed energy, health, and vigor.

You may be confronting the greatest physical challenge of your life. But with faith in God and good nutrition, combined with cutting-edge alternative natural remedies, I believe it will be your greatest victory! God revealed His divine will for each of us through the apostle John, who wrote, "Beloved, I pray that you may prosper in all things and be in health, just as your soul prospers" (3 John 2, NKJV).

Nearly two thousand years later, almost 24 million Americans suffer from a disease called diabetes—and a fourth of them don't even know they have it! Diabetes kills more people than AIDS and breast cancer combined and reportedly ranks as the sixth leading cause of death by disease among adults in America.[1] The sad reality is that it may rank much higher because research shows that diabetes is under-reported as a cause of death. Studies have found that diabetes was only listed as an underlying cause of death on 10 to 15 percent of death certificates when the decedent suffered from the disease.[2]

The World Health Organization (WHO) estimates that by 2030, the number of individuals with diabetes worldwide will double. That means we could see the number of people suffering from diabetes worldwide reach as high as 360 million within the next twenty years.[3]

Within the United States, type 2 diabetes is increasing at an alarming rate. Approximately one out of ten Americans age twenty and older has diabetes.[4] And the number of children being diagnosed with type 2 diabetes is growing at an alarming rate as well.

Researchers at the Centers for Disease Control and Prevention (CDC) recently made the stunning prediction that without changes in diet and exercise, one in three children born in the United States in 2000 are likely to develop type 2 diabetes at some point in their lives. The prediction was especially serious for Latino children, whose odds of developing diabetes as they grow older were about fifty-fifty.[5]

Why are we seeing such an increase in diabetes? It is simply the result of the obesity epidemic: two-thirds of American adults are over-weight or obese, and one-fifth of children in the United States are overweight.[6]

Surely we are missing God's best for us. But how? Many physicians are looking for the next new-and-improved medicine in order to treat diabetes. Instead, we need to get to the *root* of the problem, which is our diet, lifestyle, and waistline.

Fast food, junk food, convenience foods, sodas, sweetened coffee drinks, juices, smoothies, large portion sizes, and skipping meals are all pieces of the problem. The standard American diet is also full of empty carbohydrates, sugars, fats, excessive proteins, excessive calories, and large portion sizes, and it is quite low in nutrient content. This diet literally causes us to lose nutrients such as chromium, which is very important in glucose regulation.

Lack of activity is another piece of the problem. Most children are no longer playing sports and participating in other activities but are instead hooked on video games, computers, text messaging, TV shows, and movies as they gain more and more weight in the process.

Also, the excessive stress that most adults and many children are under is increasing cortisol levels, and, as a result, many are developing toxic belly fat, which increases the risk of diabetes. Long-term stress also depletes stress hormones as well as neurotransmitters, which usually unleash a ravenous appetite as well as addictions to sugar and carbohydrates.

DIABETES IS A "CHOICE" DISEASE

Galatians 6:7–8 says, "Do not be deceived, God is not mocked; for whatever a man sows, that he will also reap. For he who sows to his flesh will of the flesh reap corruption, but he who sows to the Spirit will of the Spirit reap everlasting life" (NKJV). Most Americans are unknowingly sowing seeds for a harvest of obesity, diabetes, and a host of other diseases by their choices of food and lifestyle habits.

I often say that prediabetes and type 2 diabetes are "choice" diseases. In other words, you *catch* a cold or you *catch* the flu, but you *develop* obesity, prediabetes, and type 2 diabetes as a result of wrong choices.

Hosea 4:6 says, "My people are destroyed for lack of knowledge" (NKJV). My books *The Seven Pillars of Health* and *Eat This and Live!* and my new weight-loss book, *Dr. Colbert's "I Can Do This" Diet*, provide a good foundation for changing dietary patterns, improving lifestyle habits, and losing weight—especially the toxic belly fat that is so closely related to diabetes.

In this book, you will learn about natural ways to avoid and reverse diabetes, but you will also learn the different types of diabetes, how it develops, and the terrible complications of diabetes as it damages and may eventually destroy the kidneys, eventually leading to dialysis. It also damages the blood vessels and may lead to blindness, impotence, heart attack, stroke, and poor circulation in the extremities. It also damages nerves, leading to burning pains in the feet (like someone is constantly burning you with cigarettes), numbness in the feet, foot and leg ulcers, infections, and possibly eventual amputation.

Now you are getting the picture as you are beginning to realize that when you habitually drink soda or eat that piece of cake, pie, candy bar, or large helping of white rice, potatoes, and white bread that you are unknowingly signing up for prediabetes and diabetes.

I have seen patients over the years stressed out over signing a contract without reading the small print. Recently, a patient came in who was very upset because after moving out of his apartment, he found out that he owed the apartment complex an extra one thousand dollars. He said that he never had to do that before after moving out of other apartments. They had informed him to simply read his contract. He did, and it said in very fine print that when the occupant of the apartment moved out, a payment of one thousand dollars would be required.

Most Americans are unknowingly signing on the dotted line for a harvest of diabetes accompanied by all of the complications associated with the disease. Wake up while there is still time to reverse the curse of diabetes and prediabetes!

You may be wondering if there is any hope, and I am here to tell you there is! You see, your body is fearfully and wonderfully made, and regardless of which type of diabetes you or a loved one may have, God can totally heal either one without effort or difficulty. I've known some people who have been completely healed of diabetes by the miracle-working power of God. I have also witnessed many others whose lives have been dramatically improved through healthy lifestyle choices and natural treatments. Realize that God generally won't do what you can do. Only you can choose to eat healthy foods, exercise, lose weight, and take supplements.

Since the original publication of *The Bible Cure for Diabetes* in 1999, many new things about diabetes have come to light, and many of the terms used to identify this illness have changed. *The New Bible Cure for Diabetes* has been revised and updated to reflect the latest medical research on diabetes. If you compare it side by side with the previous edition, you'll see that it's also larger, allowing me to expand greatly upon the information provided in the previous edition and provide you with a deeper understanding of what you face and how to overcome it.

Unchanged from the previous edition are the timeless, life-changing, and healing scriptures throughout this book that will strengthen and encourage your spirit and soul. The proven principles, truths, and guidelines in these passages anchor the practical and medical insights also contained in this book. They will effectively focus your prayers, thoughts, and actions so you can step into God's plan of divine health for you—a plan that includes victory over diabetes.

Another change since the original *The Bible Cure for Diabetes* was published is that I've released a foundational book, *The Seven Pillars of Health*. I encourage you to read it because the principles of health it contains are the foundation to healthy living that will affect all areas of your life. It sets the stage for everything you will ever read in any other book I've published—including this one.

There is much we can do to prevent or defeat diabetes. Now it is time to run to the battle with fresh confidence, renewed determination, and the wonderful knowledge that God is real, He is alive, and His power is greater than any sickness or disease.

It is my prayer that these practical suggestions for health, nutrition, and fitness will bring wholeness to your life. May they deepen your fellowship with God and strengthen your ability to worship and serve Him.

A **BIBLE CURE** *Prayer for You*

Dear heavenly Father, You have declared in Your Word that I am healed by the stripes Your Son, Jesus Christ, bore on His back. For Your Word says, "He was pierced for our rebellion, crushed for our sins. He was beaten so we could be whole. He was whipped so we could be healed" (Isa. 53:5).

Father, Your Son, Jesus, has given us the authority to use His name when we pray. This is the same name by which You spoke into being the heavens and the earth long ago. In that precious name I declare that Your Word is true: I am healed by the whipping Jesus bore on His back. Whether I must wait for a minute, a week, a year, or a lifetime for my physical healing to be complete, by faith I will praise You for it as if it were already complete. I thank You for a healthy pancreas that produces and properly regulates the insulin levels in my body. Amen.

Chapter 16

KNOW YOUR ENEMY

THOUSANDS OF YEARS ago, the Romans and Greeks had some understanding of diabetes even though they had no blood test for diabetes back then. It might surprise you to learn that the Romans and Greeks were able to detect diabetes by simply tasting a person's urine. It's true! They discovered that some people's urine had a sweet taste, or *mellitus*, which is the Latin word for "sweet." Also, the Greeks realized that when patients with sweet urine drank any fluids, the fluids were generally excreted in the urine almost as rapidly as they went in the mouth, similar to a siphon. The Greek word for "siphon" is *diabetes*. So now you know how we got the name diabetes mellitus: it all started by tasting the urine. I for one am glad that doctors abandoned this practice centuries ago and that now we simply check a patient's blood sugar!

I have good news for you too: Not only is this disease thousands of years old, but so is God's power to heal. God healed the sick thousands of years ago in the days of the Bible, and He still heals today! He has also given us a wealth of proven Bible principles and invaluable medical knowledge about the human body. You can control the symptoms and potentially damaging effects of diabetes while you seek Him for total healing. You are destined to be more than a victim. You are destined to be a victor in this battle!

Your first order of battle is to *know your enemy*. Measure its strengths, and plan for its defeat. The enemy called diabetes comes in various forms.

DIFFERENT TYPES OF DIABETES

Diabetes is actually a group of diseases including type 1 diabetes, type 2 diabetes, and gestational diabetes. Each type of diabetes is characterized by high levels of blood sugar that is the result of either defects in insulin production, defects in the action of insulin, or both.

As I said in the introduction of this book, a person does not just wake up one day with type 2 diabetes. Developing type 2 diabetes is a slow, insidious process that usually takes years to a decade to develop. It always starts with prediabetes.

Prediabetes (formerly called *borderline* or *subclinical diabetes*) is defined as a blood sugar level of 100 to 125 mg/dL (milligrams per deciliter) after an eight-hour fast. Prediabetes is also defined as a blood sugar level of 140 to 199 mg/dL two hours after eating. A normal fasting blood sugar level is less than 100 mg/dL, and a normal blood sugar level two hours after eating is less than 140 mg/dL.[1]

Diabetes is defined as a fasting blood sugar level greater than or equal to 126 mg/dL or a casual blood sugar level (usually after eating) greater than or equal to 200 mg/dL. High blood sugar levels are accompanied by symptoms of diabetes, including frequent urination, excessive thirst, and changes in vision.[2]

Type 1 diabetes

In the past, type 1 diabetes has been called insulin-dependent diabetes, juvenile-onset diabetes, or childhood-onset diabetes. This form of diabetes usually occurs in children or young adults, although it can strike at any age. In adults, it is quite rare with only about 5 to 10 percent of all cases of diabetes being type 1 diabetes.[3]

We currently do not have all the pieces of the puzzle for type 1 diabetes, but risk factors may be genetic or environmental. Some researchers believe that the environmental trigger is probably a virus. Others believe the trigger may be ingesting cow's milk protein, especially during infancy.

What we *do* know is that type 1 diabetes is caused by the body's own immune system attacking itself and eventually destroying the beta cells in the pancreas. The beta cells are the only cells in the body that make insulin, which is the hormone that regulates blood sugar.

Patients with type 1 diabetes require insulin either by injection or by an insulin pump in order to survive.

Over the years, I have found that my patients who have maintained the best blood sugar control have been the patients using the insulin pump. The newer insulin pumps actually have remote controls, making it much easier to control the blood sugar. I have also discovered that dietary and lifestyle changes and nutritional supplements will usually lower insulin requirements in type 1 diabetics. It is very important to monitor your blood sugar daily and to adjust your insulin accordingly once beginning this program. Also, have your doctor monitor you on a regular basis.

The hemoglobin A1C test is the best way to monitor your blood sugar over the long run. Hemoglobin is a protein that carries oxygen in the blood and is present inside the red blood cells that live only for about ninety to one hundred twenty days. The hemoglobin A1C measures how much glucose has entered the red blood cells and become stuck to the hemoglobin, similar to a fly stuck to flypaper.[4]

If a person usually has a high blood sugar level throughout the day, more sugar will be stuck to the hemoglobin, but if the blood sugar is typically only slightly elevated during the day, less sugar will be stuck to the hemoglobin, and the hemoglobin A1C will be lower.

Most diabetes specialists recommend that diabetic patients get their hemoglobin A1C to 6.5 percent or lower in order to prevent most of the complications of diabetes. They also recommend that the diabetic patients check this blood test approximately every three to four months. I personally try to get my diabetic patients hemoglobin A1C to around 6 percent because at this level, I find that they rarely ever develop severe complications of diabetes.

Individuals battling with type 1 diabetes will also greatly benefit from the nutritional information and biblical truths shared in this book. Continue to follow all of the advice of your physician, and consult him or her before making any lifestyle and nutritional changes. In addition, determine to believe God—who created your pancreas in the first place—for a miraculous touch of healing power. The Word of God says, "For nothing is impossible with God" (Luke 1:37).

> Don't you realize that all of you together are the temple of God and that the Spirit of God lives in you? God will destroy anyone who destroys this temple. For God's temple is holy, and you are that temple.
>
> —1 CORINTHIANS 3:16–17, NLT

Remember that faith is not a feeling or an emotion; faith is a choice. Specifically ask the Lord to heal your pancreas and restore its ability to manufacture insulin.

Type 2 diabetes

Type 2 diabetes was previously called non-insulin-dependent diabetes or adult-onset diabetes because historically people contracted the disease in their adult years. However, our nation's taste for a high-sugar, high-fat diet seems to have removed the age barrier. The medical community now reports that this form of diabetes accounts for a growing number of juvenile cases. In adults, 90 to 95 percent of all diabetes cases are type 2 diabetes. In other words, nine to nine and a half cases out of every ten cases of diabetes are type 2.[5] According to the National Institutes of Health, 1.6 million new cases of diabetes in people age twenty and older were diagnosed in 2007.[6]

Type 2 diabetes is more of a genetic disease than type 1 diabetes. However, before you blame your genes for this disease, understand this: your genetic makeup may have "loaded the gun," but environmental factors, such as belly fat, poor diet, and lifestyle factors, will "pull the trigger."

In other words, many people might have the genetic predisposition for type 2 diabetes; however, if they lose belly fat, control their diets, and exercise regularly, they will probably never develop diabetes. In fact, a large diabetes prevention study found that lifestyle changes reduced developing diabetes by more than 70 percent in high-risk people who were over sixty years old.[7]

The majority of people with type 2 diabetes still produces insulin; however, the cells in their bodies do not use the insulin properly. This condition is known as insulin resistance. Over time, insulin resistance leads to prediabetes and type 2 diabetes.

For years, I have explained to patients that insulin is like a key that unlocks the door to your cells, and having type 2 diabetes is similar to having rusty locks on those cells. Every cell in your body needs sugar, and the hormone insulin removes sugar from the bloodstream and binds to insulin receptors on the surface of the cells, very similar to a key unlocking a lock and opening the door. The insulin opens the door to the cells (figuratively speaking) and allows sugar to enter in.

However, in type 2 diabetics, the cells resist the normal function of insulin. In other words, the key goes in to unlock the lock, but, similar to a rusty lock, the insulin does not work as well. If you have ever tried to open an old, rusty lock, you will understand this analogy.

Insulin levels then begin to rise as more and more insulin is needed to allow sugar to enter into the cells. This is very similar to jiggling the key over and over until the key unlocks the rusty lock. That means that an excessive amount of insulin is needed to keep the blood sugar level in the normal range. Eventually, as cells become more and more insulin resistant, higher insulin levels are unable to lower the blood sugar. The blood sugar begins to rise higher and higher as the person develops prediabetes and eventually type 2 diabetes. Usually patients with prediabetes have no symptoms.

As this stage of insulin resistance worsens, a person will eventually develop prediabetes, which is defined as having fasting blood sugars greater than 100 mg/dL and less than 126 mg/dL. People with prediabetes typically have impaired glucose tolerance (IGT), impaired fasting glucose (IFG), or both. Often they do not know they have prediabetes because there are no symptoms initially. It typically takes years, sometimes even more than a decade, to progress from prediabetes into full-blown type 2 diabetes.

By the time people develop type 2 diabetes, they typically experience symptoms such as increased thirst, increased urination, nighttime urination, blurry vision, or fatigue. Type 2 diabetes is typically associated with obesity (especially truncal obesity), older age, a family history of diabetes, physical inactivity, or a history of gestational diabetes. Race also plays a role in risk for the disease: American Indians, Hispanic Americans, African Americans, and some Asian Americans and Pacific Islanders have a higher risk of developing type 2 diabetes and its complications.

Insulin resistance is one of the greatest health enemies of people suffering from type 2 diabetes. This is usually a very manageable problem, but it is complicated by the fact that truncal obesity is one of the most important factors leading to insulin resistance. That means that obese people with type 2 diabetes must fight a battle on two fronts: they must drop their weight down to safer levels while they also carefully monitor and control their blood sugar levels. This also means that type 2 diabetics require:

- A diet that is low in refined, processed starches such as white rice, white bread, potatoes, and pasta
- A diet that has very little sugar

A **BIBLE CURE** Health Tip

High-Fructose Corn Syrup: Sugar in Disguise

If you have diabetes, you undoubtedly have been told how important it is to limit the amount of sugar in your diet. You know you need to choose your foods carefully, but food manufacturers can be sneaky. Don't forget to watch out for one of sugar's many aliases: high-fructose corn syrup (HFCS).

HFCS is a blend of glucose and fructose. Glucose, obviously, is the form of sugar in your blood that you monitor as a diabetic. Fructose is the primary carbohydrate in most fruits. Well, if it's from fruit, it's healthy, right? Not exactly. While it is fine to consume small amounts of fructose because your body metabolizes it differently and it does not trigger your body's appetite control center, consuming large amounts sets you up for unhealthy weight gain.

Since HFCS is in many commercial food and drink products, I highly recommend that you stick to the outer aisles at the grocery store and purchase fresh produce, whole grains, and lean meats. Avoid the center aisles, and you will be well on your way to avoiding the risk of consuming a "stealth" sugar that's hidden in a packaged, processed food product. Many researchers believe that America's excessive intake of HFCS is responsible for our diabetes epidemic.

HFCS represents 40 percent of calorie sweeteners added to foods and beverages and is the only sweeteners in soft drinks in the United States. Now America consumes about sixty pounds a year of HFCS. The liver metabolizes fructose into fat more readily than it does glucose. Consuming HFCS can lead to a nonalcoholic fatty liver, which usually precedes insulin resistance and type 2 diabetes. If HFCS is one of the first ingredients on the food label, don't eat or drink it. Here is a list of foods that are high in HFCS:

- Soft drinks
- Popsicles
- Pancake syrup
- Frozen yogurt
- Breakfast cereals

- Canned fruits
- Fruit-flavored yogurt
- Ketchup and barbecue sauce
- Pasta sauces in jars and cans
- Fruit drinks that are not 100 percent fruit

Gestational diabetes

Gestational diabetes is a form of diabetes acquired during pregnancy and only occurs in about 2 percent of pregnancies. Gestational diabetes is due to the growing fetus and placenta secreting hormones that decrease the body's sensitivity to insulin and can cause diabetes.

If a woman does contract gestational diabetes, it usually goes away after giving birth. Only 5 to 10 percent of women with gestational diabetes are found to have type 2 diabetes after giving birth. However, it does increase a woman's risk of developing type 2 diabetes later in life. Studies show that 40 to 60 percent of women who developed gestational diabetes will develop type 2 diabetes within five to ten years after pregnancy. Gestational diabetes occurs more frequently among African Americans, American Indians, and Hispanic Americans.

METABOLIC SYNDROME

Many individuals who have prediabetes and type 2 diabetes also have metabolic syndrome (formerly called syndrome X). Metabolic syndrome is simply a group of risk factors, and the more of these risk factors you have, the higher your risk of heart disease, stroke, and diabetes.

You have metabolic syndrome if you have at least three of the following criteria:

- A waist measurement greater than 40 inches for men or 35 inches for women
- High blood pressure (130/85 or greater)
- Fasting blood sugar of 100 mg/dL or greater
- Triglyceride level of 150 mg/dL or greater
- Low HDL (good) cholesterol (below 40 mg/dL for men or 50 mg/dL for women)

Almost 25 percent of American adults have metabolic syndrome. Chances of developing metabolic syndrome are closely linked to overweight, obesity, and an inactive lifestyle.[8]

STRESS AND DIABETES

Excessive stress can increase glucose levels in patients with diabetes, predisposing them to long-term complications, including kidney disease, eye disease, neuropathy, and vascular disease.

In one study, diabetic patients were randomly involved in education sessions with and without stress management training. The stress management training included progressive muscle relaxation, breathing techniques, and mental imagery. All participants were at least thirty years of age and managing their diabetes with diet, exercise, and/or non-insulin medications.[9]

At the end of one year, 32 percent of the patients in the stress management group had hemoglobin A1C levels that were lowered by 1 percent or more. Hemoglobin A1C is a standard blood test used to determine average blood sugar levels over a period of a few months. Lowering hemoglobin A1C by 1 percent is considered very significant, and stress management did this in one-third of the patients. However, only 12 percent of the control subjects had hemoglobin A1C levels that were lowered by this much.[10]

Stress reduction is very important in helping to control diabetes since high cortisol levels, which is the main stress hormone, is also associated with increased belly fat, elevations of blood sugar, and increased insulin levels. I teach numerous stress-reduction techniques in my book *Stress Less*. I strongly recommend you read this book.

SYMPTOMS YOU MUST NOT IGNORE

As with most diseases, early detection of diabetes is very important. Silent enemies sometimes inflict the most damage. Fortunately, type 2 diabetes has some telltale symptoms that may tip you off to a problem that needs attention:

- Urinary frequency and nighttime urination
- Increased hunger and thirst
- Feelings of edginess, fatigue, or nausea
- Blurred vision
- Tingling, numbness, or loss of feeling in the hands or feet
- Dry, itchy skin
- Sores that don't heal
- Repeated or hard-to-heal infections of the skin, gums, vagina, or bladder
- Loss of hair on the feet and lower legs

Some of these symptoms may occur from time to time simply because you drink too much liquid one night, eat some spicy food, or stay up too late. However, if you experience one or more of these symptoms on a regular basis, make an appointment with your physician, and get screened for diabetes and prediabetes. Then you can apply the truths in this book and in God's Word to the situation. Above all, don't give in to fear or apathy.

TREATABLE AND BEATABLE

As with most diseases, serious health complications occur when someone with diabetes fails to do anything about this treatable and beatable disease. The more serious complications of diabetes include diabetic retinopathy (the leading cause of blindness in the United States), diabetic neuropathy (a degeneration of peripheral nerves that leads to tingling, numbness, pain, and weakness usually in extremities such as the legs and feet), kidney disease, and arteriosclerosis (a narrowing of the arteries due to fatty deposits on the artery walls).

> Then God said, "Look! I have given you every seed-bearing plant throughout the earth and all the fruit trees for your food. And I have given every green plant as food for all the wild animals, the birds in the sky, and the small animals that scurry along the ground—everything that has life." And that is what happened.
>
> —GENESIS 1:29–30, NLT

Diabetics—particularly those who fail to control their insulin and blood sugar levels through proper diet, exercise, and lifestyle choices—are much more prone to heart disease, heart attacks, kidney disease (one of the main causes of death in diabetics), diabetic foot ulcers (usually due to a poor blood supply), and peripheral nerve disease of the feet.

THE LONG-TERM COMPLICATIONS OF DIABETES (TERMITES)

Most people with diabetes think that they will never develop long-term complications of the disease. They rationalize that they will surely have early signs and symptoms before they develop these terrible complications of diabetes, or they assume they will be able to take medications that will reverse these diseases.

I often tell people that diabetes is very similar to a house with termites, and when termites have been eating away at a home for years, one day when you try to hang a picture on a wall, a gaping hole may suddenly appear, or your door may get stuck, and as you push on the door, the door frame may cave in. Now, this does not happen immediately with termites but with months or years of termite infestation.

Poorly controlled diabetes is a silent killer that works very similarly to termites. After years or decades, terrible health conditions suddenly begin to occur as a result of long-term diabetes. Medications can slow the process or control symptoms but usually do not get to the root of the problem.

The National Institutes of Health (NIH) say that diabetes contributes to the following diseases and health complications:

- *Vascular disease.* Individuals with poorly controlled long-term diabetes are also at a much greater risk of developing vascular disease (disease of the blood vessels). Long-term elevated blood sugar eventually accelerates plaque formation in all arteries of the body. As plaque accumulates in the coronary arteries from diabetes, people are more prone to develop heart disease or suffer a heart attack.

- Many diabetics suffer heart attacks, and due to the neuropathy, they may not experience the typical severe chest pain associated with heart attacks. Some actually experience silent heart attacks, where they feel no pain at all.

- Another type of vascular disease caused by diabetes is peripheral vascular disease, or clogging of the arteries, especially in the feet and legs. Many long-term diabetics can no longer feel their pulse in their feet, or they experience *claudication* (pain in the calves with walking that subsides with rest), both of which are symptoms of peripheral vascular disease.

- Long-term diabetics who smoke and have hypertension and high cholesterol are at a much greater risk of developing peripheral vascular disease. Fish oil, aspirin, and medications, along with aggressive risk factor modification such as blood sugar control, are usually needed to help people with peripheral vascular disease.[11]

- *Stroke.* A stroke is sometimes called a heart attack of the brain. Diabetics are very prone to plaque buildup in the arteries that supply blood to the brain, putting them at an increased risk of stroke. A diabetic may have a TIA (transient ischemic attack) in which he develops slurring of the speech, numbness, or weakness on one side of the body that usually goes away after a few hours. Having a TIA is a very ominous sign of an impending stroke, and you should go to the emergency room or see your physician immediately if you experience this.[12]

- *High blood pressure.* An estimated 73 percent of adults with diabetes also have high blood pressure or are taking medications for hypertension.[13] The cause should be obvious, considering the effects of diabetes on the cardiovascular and circulatory system mentioned earlier.

- *Eye disease.* Long-term diabetes also affects the eyes and may lead to diabetic retinopathy, loss of vision, and eventual blindness. Diabetic retinopathy is a common condition seen in diabetics who have had the disease for more than ten years. Between 40 and 45 percent of people with diabetes have some stage of diabetic retinopathy.[14] Diabetic retinopathy causes up to twenty-four thousand new cases of blindness every year.[15]

- Without good blood sugar control, numerous changes occur in the eyes that can be seen on the retina of the eyes. Diabetes causes a weakening of the tiny blood vessels in the eyes, and they may eventually rupture and form retinal hemorrhages. These hemorrhages can form clots that may eventually cause retinal detachment.

- If you are diabetic, it is very important that an ophthalmologist examines you annually. An ophthalmologist will examine the eyes, thoroughly checking for signs of retinopathy. He may decide to use laser surgery to save your vision, but as a result of laser surgery, some may have minor loss of vision as well as a decrease in night vision. This is why it is critically important to maintain good blood sugar control if diabetic retinopathy is detected.

- *Kidney disease.* In the United States, diabetes is the underlying cause of approximately half of the people who require long-term dialysis, as well as being the leading cause of kidney failure.[16]

- However, don't let these statistics scare you. The majority of people with diabetes do *not* develop kidney disease, and of those who do, most do not progress to kidney failure. This is good news. It means that even with diabetes, simply controlling your blood sugar will almost always prevent kidney disease.

- Controlling your blood sugar and blood pressure, along with maintaining a healthy diet and losing weight, is critically important if you are facing the challenge of kidney disease. Your doctor may prescribe a medication such as an ACE inhibitor, and I recommend a form of vitamin B$_6$, which also helps to protect the kidneys. You will learn more about this in chapter 20.

- Kidney failure can be avoided if kidney disease is detected early on. But the early stages of kidney disease usually remain undetected with a regular urinalysis. Therefore, it's important to get a specific test for microalbumin that can detect protein in the urine years before a regular urinalysis can. Make sure your doctor checks the microalbumin level in your urine annually at least.

- *Diabetic neuropathy.* Long-term diabetes eventually affects the nerves, leading to diabetic neuropathy. Approximately 60 to 70 percent of diabetics have some form of peripheral nerve damage, which often affects the feet and hands, and the patient usually describes symptoms of numbness or decreased ability to feel light touch and pain.[17] They also usually develop burning and tingling or extreme sensitivity to touch, especially in their feet, and their symptoms are usually worse at night.

- Diabetic neuropathy may eventually lead to foot ulcers. Sometimes these foot ulcers become infected, and if not treated promptly, they may lead to severe infection and eventual amputation. Maintaining good foot care, wearing comfortable shoes and socks, carefully inspecting your feet daily, and maintaining good blood sugar control are very important in treating diabetic neuropathy. Also, I recommend to my diabetic patients to never go outdoors barefoot.

- I also recommend that people with diabetic neuropathy see a podiatrist or foot specialist on a regular basis. In chapter 20, you will find great nutritional supplements that are usually very effective in helping diabetic neuropathy.

- *Amputations.* More than half of lower-limb amputations in the United States occur among people with diabetes. In recent years, this number has been as high as seventy-one thousand lower-limb amputations per year being performed on people with diabetes.[18] The lower extremities are more susceptible to the circulatory impairment caused by diabetes simply because they are further from the heart. The nutrients and oxygen in the bloodstream must make their way through a much greater distance of blood vessels and capillaries to nourish cells in the feet and toes.

- *Dental disease.* Dental disease, in the form of periodontal disease (a type of gum disease that can lead to tooth loss), occurs with greater frequency and severity among people with diabetes. People with poorly controlled diabetes are three times more likely to develop severe periodontitis than those without diabetes.[19]

- *Pregnancy complications.* Poorly controlled diabetes prior to conception and during the first three months of pregnancy can cause major birth defects and even spontaneous abortion. During the second and third trimesters, if diabetes is not controlled, it can result in large babies, posing a risk to both mother and child.[20]

- *Other illnesses.* Diabetics are also more susceptible to other illnesses and have a worse prognosis if they do come down with these illnesses. For instance, diabetics are more likely to die from flu and pneumonia than nondiabetics.[21]

- *Erectile dysfunction.* A very common complication of diabetes is impotence or erectile dysfunction, which is the inability to have or sustain an erection sufficient for intercourse. It is estimated that 50 to 60 percent of diabetic men over the age of fifty will experience erectile dysfunction.[22] However, if discovered early enough, this can be prevented or even reversed by losing belly fat, controlling blood sugar with diet and exercise, stress reduction, and taking supplements and hormone replacement.

THE GOOD NEWS

After reading through all of these dismal complications, you may feel like tiny David when he stood before the nine-foot giant called Goliath. Don't give in to fear. These are the complications that most often affect diabetics whose blood sugar levels are not controlled through proper diet and exercise.

In the face of these medical facts, your goal is to take advantage of the wealth of wisdom in God's Word and in the medical knowledge He has given us over the centuries to avoid these complications altogether by making wise choices. Most importantly, your primary goal is to take hold of the healing Jesus offers you.

A **BIBLE CURE** Prayer for You

Dear heavenly Father, help me make wise choices and follow the guidelines in Your Word concerning food choices, lifestyle, prayer, and a thought life that is saturated with Your living Word. Thank You for hearing and answering my prayer so I will be free to serve You with my whole mind, body, soul, and strength. Amen.

A **BIBLE CURE** *Prescription*

Faith Builder

> But he was pierced for our rebellion, crushed for our sins. He was beaten so we could be whole. He was whipped so we could be healed.
>
> —ISAIAH 53:5, NLT

Write out this verse, and insert your own name into it: "He was pierced for _____'s rebellion, He was crushed for _____'s sins; He was beaten so that _____ could be made whole and whipped so that _____ could be healed!"

Write out a personal prayer to Jesus Christ, thanking Him for exchanging His health for your pain. Thank Him for taking the power of sickness onto His own body so that He could purchase your healing from diabetes.

_____

_____

_____

_____

_____

_____

_____

_____

_____

_____

_____

_____

_____

_____

Chapter 17

BATTLE DIABETES WITH GOOD NUTRITION

THE SAME GOD who skillfully designed your body as an incredible, living creation and created your pancreas to produce insulin also designed the human body to operate at peak efficiency and health when it is supplied with proper nutrition. If you are a diabetic, what you eat makes all the difference in the world!

Ask God to give you a new way of looking at nutrition. You'll be surprised at the way your thinking about food begins to change. First, and most importantly, you must stop looking at the scale and start looking at your waistline as a key indicator of weight management.

YOUR WAISTLINE IS YOUR LIFELINE

Why wait until you have a major complication like the list we covered at the end of chapter 16 before you start controlling your blood sugar? Take a proactive approach to diabetes by first realizing that your waistline is your lifeline. If your waist measurement increases, your blood sugar will typically increase, and if your waist measurement decreases, your blood sugar will typically decrease. By focusing on your waistline and following a doctor's plan and exercise advice to shrink your waist, you will find that your blood sugar will lower according to your waist measurement.

Let's start with an understanding of how to measure your waist. Over the years, I've discovered that many men do not measure their waists correctly. They may have a 52-inch waist, but they don't realize it because they still fit into jeans with a 32-inch waist. Their huge bellies are hanging over their belts, and yet they are adamant that they have a 32-inch waist.

Also, over the last several years, low-waisted pants have become popular in many women's clothing styles. As a result, I have seen more and more women measuring too low for their waist measurement as well.

Your waist is measured around your belly button (and around your love handles if you have them). I have had patients who were shocked by the reality of their true waist measurement once I showed them the proper place to measure. As the reality sinks in, I help them devise the following plan to reach their waist measurement goal.

First, put away your scale since daily or weekly weighing usually leads to disappointment, and you may eventually give up. Instead, follow your waist measurement on a monthly basis.

Second, establish a waist measurement goal. Initially, the waist measurement goal for a man with diabetes or prediabetes is 40 inches or less. For a woman with prediabetes or diabetes the goal is to have a waist measurement of 35 inches or less.

Third, take your height in inches and divide it by two. Eventually, your waist measurement should be equal to this number or less. In other words, your waist should measure half of your height or less. For example, a 5-foot-8-inch man would be 68 inches tall, so his waist should be 34 inches or less around the belly button and love handles.

Notice that this is the *third* step, especially for prediabetics and type 2 diabetics. Decrease your waist to 40 inches or less (for men) or 35 inches or less (for women) before you worry about getting it down to half your height or less.

I can promise you that you will be amazed as your blood sugar drops with every inch lost in your waist.

WHAT IS THE GLYCEMIC INDEX?

The glycemic index gives an indication of the rate at which different carbs break down to release sugar into the bloodstream. More precisely, it assesses a numeric value to how rapidly the blood sugar rises after consuming a food that contains carbohydrates. Keep in mind the fact that the glycemic index is only for carbohydrates and not for fats or proteins.

Sugars and carbohydrates that are digested rapidly, such as white bread, white rice, and instant potatoes, raise the blood sugar rapidly. These are considered high-glycemic foods because they have a glycemic index of 70 or higher. If the glycemic index for a certain food is high, then it will raise your blood sugar levels much faster (this is bad). High blood sugar levels, in turn, increase the amount of insulin that will be secreted by type 2 diabetics and prediabetics to bring the blood sugar level back into balance.

> Don't worry about anything; instead, pray about everything. Tell God what you need, and thank him for all he has done. Then you will experience God's peace, which exceeds anything we can understand. His peace will guard your hearts and minds as you live in Christ Jesus.
>
> —Philippians 4:6–7, NLT

On the other hand, if foods containing carbohydrates are digested slowly and therefore release sugars gradually or slowly into the bloodstream, they have a low glycemic index value of 55 or lower. These foods include most vegetables and fruits, beans, peas, lentils, sweet potatoes, and the like. Because these foods cause the blood sugar to rise more slowly, insulin levels do not rise significantly and the blood sugar levels are stabilized for a longer period of time. Low-glycemic foods also cause satiety hormones to be released in the small intestines, which keeps you satisfied longer.

As an example of the various glycemic index values for different foods, glucose has a value of 100, while broccoli and cabbage, both of which contain little or no carbohydrates, have a value of 0 to 1. In truth, there is nothing fancy about the glycemic index. One of the most important factors that can determine the food's glycemic index value is simply how much the food has been processed. Generally speaking, the more highly processed a food, the higher its glycemic index value; the more natural a food, the lower its glycemic index value.

A **BIBLE CURE** *Health Tip*

Rule of Thumb: The Glycemic Index

Low-glycemic foods are 55 or less.

Medium-glycemic foods are 56 to 69.

High-glycemic foods are 70 and above.

THE GLYCEMIC LOAD

Almost twenty years after the glycemic index was established as a standard of measurement, researchers at Harvard University developed a new way of classifying foods that took into account not only the glycemic index value of a food but also the quantity of carbohydrates that food contains. This is called the glycemic load (GL). It gives us a guide as to how much quantity of a particular carbohydrate or food we should eat.

For a while, nutritionists scratched their heads as patients desiring to lose weight were eating low-glycemic foods yet were not losing weight. In fact, some were actually gaining weight. The problem, they discovered through the GL, was that overconsuming many types of low-glycemic foods can actually lead to weight gain. And these patients were eating as many low-glycemic foods as they wanted, simply because they had been told that foods with a low glycemic index value were better for weight loss.

You can determine the glycemic load of a food by multiplying the glycemic index value by the quantity of carbohydrates a serving contains (in grams), and then dividing that number by 100. The actual formula looks like this:

(*Glycemic index value x carb grams per serving*) / 100 = *glycemic load*

To show you how important the GL is, let me offer some examples. Some wheat pastas have a low glycemic index value, which makes many dieters think they're an automatic key to losing weight. However, if a serving size of that wheat pasta is too large, it may sabotage your weight loss efforts because, despite a low glycemic index value, the GL is high. On the other extreme, watermelon has a high glycemic index value but a very low GL, which makes it OK to eat in a larger quantity. Yet another example, the GL of white potatoes is double that of sweet potatoes.

> You must serve only the LORD your God. If you do, I will bless you with food and water, and I will protect you from illness.
> —EXODUS 23:25, NLT

Don't worry, I am not recommending that you calculate the GL for every item at every meal you eat. The main point is that by understanding the GL, you can identify which low-glycemic foods can cause trouble if you eat too much of them. These include low-glycemic breads, low-glycemic rice, sweet potatoes, low-glycemic pasta, and low-glycemic cereals. As a general rule, any large quantity of a low-glycemic "starchy" food will usually have a high GL, so limit the serving to no larger than a tennis ball.

Keep in mind also that if you use the GL without considering the glycemic index, you will probably be eating more of an Atkins-type diet with lots of fats and proteins and very few carbohydrates—which is not a healthy way to eat in the long run and can cause insulin resistance.

A BIBLE CURE Health Tip

Glycemic Index Values of Common Foods[1]

To look up the glycemic index values of other foods not listed here, go to www.glycemicindex.com.

Food	Glycemic Index Value
Asparagus	<15
Broccoli	<15
Celery	<15
Cucumber	<15
Green beans	<15
Lettuce (all varieties)	<15
Low-fat yogurt (artificially sweetened)	<15
Peppers (all varieties)	<15

Food	Glycemic Index Value
Spinach	<15
Zucchini	<15
Tomatoes	15
Cherries	22
Milk (skim)	32
Spaghetti (whole wheat)	37
Apples	38
All-Bran cereal	42
Lentil soup (tinned)	44
Whole-grain bread	50
Orange juice	52
Bananas	54
Potato (sweet)	54
Rice (brown)	55
Popcorn	55
Muesli	56
Whole-meal bread	69
Watermelon	72
Doughnut	76
Rice cakes	77
Corn Flakes	83
Potato (baked)	85
Baguette	95
Parsnips	97
Dates	103

Additional foods with high glycemic index levels that you need to limit or avoid include instant potatoes, instant rice, French bread, white bread, corn, processed oats, instant potatoes, white rice, most boxed cereals (such as cornflakes), baked potatoes, mashed potatoes, cooked carrots, honey, raisins, dried fruit, candy bars, crackers, cookies, ice cream, and pastries. If you are diabetic, you should either eat these foods very rarely or avoid them completely.

Remember that high-glycemic foods and high-density carbohydrates raise blood sugar quickly, which in turn raises insulin levels. When this occurs long term, the high insulin levels cause your cells to become resistant to insulin. You might say that these high-glycemic foods are similar to a toxin in an individual with type 2 diabetes.

> If you will listen carefully to the voice of the LORD your God and do what is right in his sight, obeying his commands and keeping all his decrees, then I will not make you suffer any of the diseases I sent on the Egyptians; for I am the LORD who heals you.
>
> —EXODUS 15:26, NLT

If you are dealing with type 2 diabetes, your pancreas may be producing about four times as much insulin as a nondiabetic's pancreas. The key to correcting your cells' resistance to insulin is following the proper diet. You must decrease or avoid sugars and high-glycemic starches, such as breads, white rice, potatoes, and corn, and decrease fats, including saturated fats, and fried foods. If you will do this, your cells will eventually recover. They will begin to regain their sensitivity to insulin. You hold the key.

THE BIBLE AND FATS

Interestingly, eating certain fats is condemned in the Bible. God commands, "You must never eat any fat or blood. This is a permanent law for you, and it must be observed from generation to generation, wherever you live" (Lev. 3:17, NLT). This verse is referring to the toxic belly fat of the animal, which also includes the fat around the kidneys and liver. The fat in this verse is also translated "grease." God created our bodies and knows how they have been designed to function best. I encourage you to substitute a small amount of extra-virgin olive oil and flaxseed oil as well as other healthy oils for butter, cream, and other fats. Do not cook with flaxseed oil. Always choose low-fat portions of meat as well. Especially avoid trans fats, hydrogenated fats, and partially hydrogenated fats. Excessive amounts of saturated fats and any trans fats are associated with insulin resistance. For more information on this topic, refer to *The Seven Pillars of Health.*

A **BIBLE CURE** *Health Tip*

Antidiabetogenic Foods

Gabriel Cousens, MD, author of *There Is a Cure for Diabetes*, recommends the following foods for their therapeutic properties in the treatment of diabetes.[2]

- Jerusalem artichoke—an herbal medicine that contains inulin, which prevents your blood sugar from rising rapidly.

- Bitter melon—a green tropical fruit that resembles a cucumber and contains several antidiabetic properties.

- Cucumber—contains a hormone your pancreas needs to produce insulin.

- Celery—has general antidiabetogenic qualities and also helps lower your blood pressure, which is a symptom of metabolic syndrome.

- Garlic and onion—contain sulfur compounds believed to be the reason for their antidiabetic effects.

- Walnuts—a handful contains high amounts of monounsaturated fat, omega-3 fatty acid, and alpha linolenic acid (ALA), which help to lower cholesterol and fats in your blood and are important in protecting against diabetes.

- Almonds—a handful provides vitamin E, magnesium, and fiber. *The Journal of Nutrition* reported that almonds and walnuts provide glycemic control when you add them to a high-carbohydrate meal.

- Kelp—this sea vegetable promotes thyroid health, and your thyroid controls your metabolism, which in turn affects your ability to lose weight.

FANTASTIC FIBER

Another important way you can battle diabetes through nutrition is to increase the fiber in your diet. Dietary fiber is extremely important in helping to control diabetes. Fiber slows down digestion and the absorption of carbohydrates. This allows for a more gradual rise in blood sugar.

If you have diabetes, a significant amount of the carbohydrate calories you eat should come from vegetables, including peas, beans, lentils, and legumes. Those vegetables typically contain large amounts of fiber. The more soluble fiber in your diet, the better blood sugar control your body will have.

> That is why I tell you not to worry about everyday life—whether you have enough food and drink, or enough clothes to wear. Isn't life more than food, and your body more than clothing? Look at the birds. They don't plant or harvest or store food in barns, for your heavenly Father feeds them. And aren't you far more valuable to him than they are?
>
> —MATTHEW 6:25–26, NLT

Water-soluble fibers are found in oat bran, seeds such as psyllium (the primary ingredient in Metamucil), fruit and vegetables (especially apples and pears), beans, and nuts. You should try to take in at least 30 to 35 g of fiber a day. You also should take the fiber with meals in order to prevent rapid rises in blood sugar.

A **BIBLE CURE** *Health Tip*

Increasing Fiber in Your Diet

You might try the following ideas to increase the fiber in your diet:

1. Eat at least five servings of fruit and vegetables each day. Fruit and vegetables that are high in fiber include:

- Granny Smith apples
- Peas
- Broccoli
- Spinach
- Berries
- Pears

- Brussels sprouts
- Beans (all types)
- Parsnips
- Legumes
- Carrots (not cooked)
- Lentils

2. Replace breads and cereals made from refined flours with whole-grain breads and cereals. Eat brown rice instead of white rice. Examples of these foods include:

- Walnuts, almonds, and macadamia nuts

- Old-fashioned steel-cut oatmeal or high-fiber instant oatmeal

- Brown rice

- Flaxseeds, chia seeds, hemp seeds, pumpkin seeds, and sunflower seeds

- Ezekiel bread or other sprouted bread

3. Eat high-fiber cereal for breakfast. Check labels on the packages for the amounts of dietary fiber in each brand. Some cereals may have less fiber than you think. Fiber One cereal, Kashi Cinnamon Harvest, and Kashi Island Vanilla are good choices

4. Eat cooked beans, peas, or lentils a few times a week.

5. Take PGX fiber (two to three capsules with 16 oz. of water before each meal.

Many foods contain dietary fiber. Eating foods that are high in fiber can not only help relieve some problems with diabetes but also may help lower your cholesterol and even prevent heart disease and certain types of cancer.

A WORD OF CAUTION

When adding fiber to your diet, make small changes over a period of time to help prevent bloating, cramping, or gas. Start by adding one of the items listed above to your diet, then wait several days or even a week before making another change. If one change doesn't seem to work for you, try a different one.

It's important to drink more fluids when you increase the amount of fiber you eat. Drink at least two additional glasses of water a day when you increase your fiber intake.

This information provides a general overview on dietary fiber and may not apply to everyone. I have included some advice in chapter 19 and chapter 20 to help you increase your fiber intake through diet and nutritional supplements. I also recommend reading my book *Dr. Colbert's "I Can Do This" Diet*.

A **BIBLE CURE** Health Tip

Avoid Soy

For the last few years I have been warning people about the use of soy because I've seen many people have adverse reactions to consuming it. Others in the medical community are beginning to speak out as well.

Gabriel Cousens, MD, calls soy a *diabetogenic* food, meaning it produces diabetes. Cousens explains that 90 percent of all soy is genetically modified (GMO). Soy is also one of the top seven allergens. The isoflavones in soy can make a person estrogenic, contributing to cancer of the breast, and uterine fibroids. Cousens also links soy to decreased thyroid production, stunted growth in children, lowering of good (HDL) cholesterol, insulin resistance, heart disease, and Alzheimer's disease.[3]

WHAT ABOUT BREAD?

Americans love white bread, coffee, and hot dogs. However, processing white bread removes all the bran and germ, along with approximately 80 percent of the nutrients and virtually all the fiber. Bleaching the flour destroys even more vitamins. Sugar and hydrogenated fats are added, right along with manufactured vitamins. In the end you get a product that is pure starch—stripped of the fiber and nutritional value of whole-grain breads. Add water to white bread, and it forms a sticky, glue-like substance. Is there any wonder why this food takes double the amount of time to be eliminated from the body?

America's romance with processed foods, such as breads, potatoes, and other grains, is one of the main reasons we see diabetes increasing every year at alarming rates.

> I know how to live on almost nothing or with everything. I have learned the secret of living in every situation, whether it is with a full stomach or empty, with plenty or little. For I can do everything through Christ, who gives me strength.
> —PHILIPPIANS 4:12–13, NLT

Today the best choices of bread are the sprouted breads found in most health food stores. I personally choose Ezekiel bread, which is made of the sprouts of wheat, barley, and other grains.

Remember, even if breads at the supermarket are called whole-grain breads, they also may contain sugar and hydrogenated fats and are processed in such a way that they still have fairly high glycemic indexes. Therefore, if my diabetic patients request bread, I recommend that they have moderate amounts of sprouted bread, such as Ezekiel bread, in the morning or at lunch. I find that it tastes better when toasted. You can find Ezekiel bread in many grocery stores in the frozen food section and online. Try it. You'll love the taste! The new double-fiber breads are a step in the right direction, but I still prefer the sprouted breads.

A **BIBLE CURE** Health Fact

Coffee Lowers Risk of Developing Diabetes

Three different studies have shown that coffee consumption helps decrease the risk of developing type 2 diabetes. An analysis of over seventeen thousand Dutch men and women found that the more coffee a person drinks, the lower the risk for developing type 2 diabetes. Consuming three to four cups of coffee a day decreased the risk of developing diabetes by 23 percent, and people who drank over seven cups a day cut their risk in half.[4]

A Finnish study found that consuming three to four cups of coffee a day decreased type 2 diabetes risk by 24 percent, and consuming ten or more cups a day lowered the risk by 61 percent.[5]

Another study of coffee consumption explored the benefits of caffeinated versus decaffeinated coffee. Men who drank one to three cups of decaf coffee a day decreased their risk of diabetes by 9 percent while those who drank four or more cups a day lowered it by 26 percent.[6]

Please note that these studies pertain to *preventing* diabetes. More studies are needed before we can conclusively state the effects of coffee in people who are already diabetic. Some studies have shown that excessive caffeine raises blood sugar, and unfortunately, most Americans consume their coffee loaded with sugar and cream that are likely to raise blood sugar as well. For this reason, I do not advise people with diabetes to drink more than one or two cups of organic coffee (sweetened with stevia) per day.

If you are interested in preventing diabetes, an alternative to drinking coffee is taking coffee berry extract. Coffee berry is the fruit that produces coffee beans. The powerful *phytonutrients* that quench free radicals and help manage blood sugar are found in the whole fruit and not just the bean. I generally recommend 100 mg of coffee berry extract, three times a day.

A FINAL WORD

In summary, proper diet is still the cornerstone for treating diabetes. If you are a type 1 diabetic, you must avoid sugar altogether and dramatically limit starches. Limit fruit as well, because it can also raise your blood sugar dramatically. High-fiber foods such as legumes (beans) and root vegetables (uncooked carrots) will help to lower your blood sugar. Type 1 diabetics must also avoid fruit juices. Your physician or dietician should closely monitor your diet.

However, if you are a type 2 diabetic, you can benefit from small amounts of low-glycemic fruit that is high in fiber, such as pears and Granny Smith apples, if they are used conservatively. Do not drink fruit juice or eat applesauce.

The most important dietary advice is to avoid sugar and to dramatically limit refined starches, including white breads, refined pasta, potatoes, most cereals, white rice, and other highly processed foods.

A **BIBLE CURE** Prayer for You

Dear heavenly Father, You are the One who will help me throughout my life if I let You. You don't expect me to be perfect, just to receive You into my life. When I've blown it in the way I eat and the way I live, You are ready to forgive and help me to stay on course. Your power to forgive is as great as Your power to love. I will never forget how much You love me. Amen.

A **BIBLE CURE** Prescription

Toward a New Nutritional Lifestyle

List the top five problem foods that you crave and that have a high GI:

_____

_____

_____

_____

_____

List five healthy food choices you will make this week instead:

_____

_____

_____

_____

_____

In what ways do you need God's help to change your eating habits?

_____

_____

_____

Write out a Bible cure prayer asking for God's help in making these changes.

_____

_____

_____

_____

Chapter 18

BATTLE DIABETES WITH ACTIVITY

YOUR BODY, THE dwelling place of God's Spirit, needs to be protected and kept healthy. Remember, your body was bought by the blood of Jesus, and you are to glorify God in your body and in your spirit (1 Cor. 6:20, NKJV). You must do your part, which involves choosing the correct foods and beverages and exercising the body on a regular basis. You must take courage and continually battle diabetes because it can weaken and damage other organs in your body.

I cannot stress enough how important it is to overcome your diabetes with exercise. Exercise holds special benefits for diabetics. Multiple studies have shown that those who have a physically active lifestyle are less prone to develop type 2 diabetes. I believe this is because physical exercise battles the root of type 2 diabetes, which gets its start when muscle cells lose their sensitivity to insulin. Research has shown that your muscle cells are much less likely to become resistant to insulin if you keep them fit through regular exercise.

Studies have also shown that regular exercise improves glucose tolerance and lowers blood sugar as well as insulin requirements. The more muscle tissue that we develop in our large muscle groups such as the thighs and buttocks, the more sugar will be removed from the bloodstream. The greater the muscle mass in especially the large muscle groups is likely associated with a corresponding drop in insulin resistance. Also, by burning calories, exercise helps control weight, an important factor in the management of type 2 diabetes.

A study at the Cooper Institute for Aerobics Research in Dallas shows that staying fit may be the most important thing you can do to avoid type 2 diabetes. The researchers put 8,633 men with an average age of forty-three through a treadmill test and then screened them for diabetes six years later. The men who scored poorly on the fitness test were almost four times more likely to have developed the disease than those who had done well on the treadmill. In fact, the fitness scores turned out to be the most accurate predictor of diabetes—more than age, obesity, high blood pressure, or family history of the disease.[1]

A **BIBLE CURE** Health Tip

Important!

Before undergoing any activity or fitness program, please check with your doctor to make sure that you are healthy enough to participate.

If you don't participate in at least thirty minutes of exercise per day, talk with your doctor about ways to incorporate more exercise into your everyday life. Because I'm a doctor and have advised many patients over the years, I know that most people immediately visualize exercise as just another chore, or they think it will be embarrassing, draining, or very unpleasant. So instead of exercise, let's simply think of this as "increasing your activity level." Here are a few quick tips to get you started:

- First, you need to choose an activity that is fun and enjoyable. You will never stick to any activity program if you dread or hate it.

- Also, I find it is best to do your activity program with a friend or partner.

- Make sure that you wear comfortable, well-fitting shoes and socks.

- If you are a type 1 diabetic, you will need to work with your doctor in order to adjust your insulin doses while increasing your activity. Realize that exercising will lower your blood sugar; this can be potentially dangerous in a type 1 diabetic.

Now, let's discuss the different types of activities you can choose from.

AEROBIC ACTIVITY

Examples of aerobic activity are walking, cycling, swimming, working out on an elliptical machine, dancing, and hiking; it's any movement that raises the heart rate enough to help you burn fat. I used to have patients figure out their training heart rate zone and keep their heart rate in that zone. This is certainly good to do, and with new aerobic exercise equipment, one simply holds onto the handles and the machine calculates your heart rate for you. However, I've found that most diabetics hate going to a gym and simply will not exercise. For them, I recommend the perceived exertion scale.

A **BIBLE CURE** *Health Tip*

Perceived Exertion Scale

This is a scale that ranks your perceived exertion as:

1. Very, very light
2. Very light
3. Fairly light
4. Somewhat hard
5. Very hard
6. Very, very hard

Usually, when you exercise at a perceived exertion of somewhat hard, you are typically in your target heart rate zone.

One of the best aerobic activities is simply brisk walking. A very simple way to enter your target heart rate zone is to simply walk briskly enough so that you cannot sing and slowly enough so that you can talk. This simple formula works for most of my patients. If you are walking so slow that you can sing, simply speed up. But if you are walking so fast that you cannot talk, then slow down. This is another reason why you need an activity partner or buddy to talk with as you walk.

For diabetic patients with foot ulcers or numbness in the feet, walking is not the best activity for you. Instead, try cycling, the elliptical machine, or pool activities. Be sure to inspect your feet well before and after your activity session.

If you are able to walk, simply walk in your neighborhood or a nearby park, starting with a five- or ten-minute walk, and increase it gradually as tolerated. Many of my patients eventually prefer to walk for ten to fifteen minutes in the morning after breakfast and ten to fifteen minutes in the evening after dinner.

By breaking up the activity program into two shorter time segments, most people find it easier to handle. Simply walking your dog twice a day will usually do the trick. It is also good to walk as a family after dinner and use the time to connect with each other, laugh, and unwind.

RESISTANCE EXERCISES

Resistance training usually involves lifting weights to build muscles. I have shared this simple rule of thumb with my diabetic patients for years: the more muscle you build in the lower extremities and buttocks, generally the better blood sugar control you will have.

> While dining with a ruler, pay attention to what is put before you. If you are a big eater, put a knife to your throat; don't desire all the delicacies, for he might be trying to trick you.
> —PROVERBS 23:1–3, NLT

Scientific studies have proven that a combination of resistance training and aerobic exercise is the most effective way to improve insulin sensitivities in diabetics.[2] That is why I call aerobic activity and resistance training a one-two punch to knock out type 2 diabetes.

Aerobic activity combined with resistance training will improve blood sugar control even better than most diabetic medications.

I usually start patients with simple resistance exercises like those I describe in my book *The Seven Pillars of Health* and eventually graduate them to resistance exercises with weights. I strongly recommend starting with a certified personal trainer in order to instruct you in the proper technique and to develop a good resistance program with emphasis on increasing strength and muscle mass in the lower extremities.

Over time, I find that most diabetics benefit from activity five days a week, with at least thirty to forty-five minutes of aerobic activity and fifteen to thirty minutes of resistance exercises three times a week. Remember, this one-two punch of resistance training and aerobic activity is better than medication for diabetes.

STICKING WITH IT

Many people find that, difficult as it is to start an exercise program, it is even more difficult to stick with it. Too many people get into trouble when they save exercising for their spare time. If you wait until you can get around to it, you probably never will. Make exercise a priority as important as a doctor's appointment.

> Do you like honey? Don't eat too much, or it will make you sick!...It's not good to eat too much honey.
> —PROVERBS 25:16, 27, NLT

Choose an exercise activity that you truly enjoy. Walking is only one suggestion. Have you tried ballroom dancing? Or backpacking? Perhaps you've always pictured yourself on a tennis court. Surely there is an activity that you always thought you'd like to try. Now's the time—try it. If you enjoy it, then stick with it.

In addition, most people feel calm and have a sense of well-being after they exercise. You can actually walk off your anxieties. Exercise releases endorphins, which are morphine-like substances that give us feelings of well-being. People who exercise feel better about themselves, look better, feel more energetic, and are more productive at work.

NOW, TAKE THE OFFENSIVE!

Take the offensive, and follow the positive steps suggested in this chapter. You will discover how effective God's wisdom can be in both the spiritual and natural realms. God heals in many ways, whether through supernatural means or through the more gradual—but equally divine—means of proper nutrition, exercise, and biblical life choices.

A **BIBLE CURE** *Prayer for You*

Lord, help me to change my habits. I need Your strength and deter-
mination when mine weakens. Give me the desire and motivation
I need to succeed. Lord Jesus, I choose to believe that the power
of the cross is greater than my bondage to diabetes. You love me
and died on the cross to free me from all of my bondages. I crucify
my flesh daily and choose to give it what it needs and not what
it craves. I now know it needs exercise and increased activity. I,
(your name), *choose faith today,* (date). *I give You these* (how many
pounds) *pounds—and confess by faith that I weigh* _____ *pounds*
(define goal). *In Jesus's name I declare victory today! Amen.*

A **BIBLE CURE** *Prescription*

Battling Diabetes With Exercise

What activity or exercise are you getting at least five days a week?

_____

_____

_____

How are you monitoring your heart rate?

_____

_____

_____

What are your goals for increasing the amount of activity or exercise you get regularly?

_____

_____

_____

Think about what partner you will choose to be your exercise buddy—your neighbor, friend, spouse, child, etc.

_____

_____

_____

What time is best to make in your schedule to have a consistent exercise time? Your exercise time should be viewed as important as a doctor's appointment.

_____

_____

_____

Chapter 19

BATTLE DIABETES WITH WEIGHT LOSS

Have you been battling a weight problem all of your life with little or no success? No one has to tell you that many cases of diabetes are directly linked to obesity. Determine right now that, with God's help, you will get to your ideal weight and stay there. Perhaps you've been overweight for so long that you've given up. In the back of your mind you may even be thinking, "It's impossible for me to lose weight."

The Bible says, "Nothing is impossible with God." (See Luke 1:37, NKJV.) It may seem virtually impossible for you alone. But you are not alone! God is on your side, and His strength is available to help you.

Don't even try to face this issue alone. You don't have to. At this moment, whisper a prayer with me asking God to strengthen you to overcome any sense of defeat and bondage that obesity has caused in your life.

A Powerful Key to Prevention

Weight control is a powerful key to the reversal and the prevention of diabetes. Type 2 diabetes is directly linked to obesity and diets rich in sugars, refined carbohydrates, and fats. Since it is far better to prevent diabetes altogether rather than to reverse the disease and ask God to heal you afterward, I strongly encourage you to lose weight if necessary if you are seeking to prevent diabetes. If you already have type 2 diabetes, weight control is absolutely essential.

Your Ideal Weight—Catch the Vision!

Close your eyes, and picture yourself walking around in the body that God intended for you to have—the healthy one. You don't have to shop in plus-size stores anymore. You move easily and confidently and no longer huff and puff when you climb stairs. You will wear a bathing suit with comfort and confidence. Are you catching the vision?

It is absolutely essential that you see yourself weighing a healthy weight on a daily basis and place a picture of yourself at a healthy weight around the house, on your vanity mirror, or on your fridge. Then confess daily that you weigh your desired weight by faith.

As you visualize yourself weighting a certain weight or being a certain size and confess it daily, you reset your mental autopilot, and you will start to lose weight. Do not say, "I will lose 30 or 40 pounds by faith," or else you will always have 30 or 40 pounds to lose.

> So whether you eat or drink, or whatever you do, do it all for the glory of God.
>
> —1 CORINTHIANS 10:31, NLT

Write down your desired weight in the space provided.

My desired weight is _____ pounds.

My actual weight is _____ pounds.

I need to lose _____ pounds.

Realize that your waist measurement is more important than your weight. Remember, your eventual goal is a waist measurement of less than half of your height.

A **BIBLE CURE** *Health Fact*

BMI, Waist Size, and Type 2 Diabetes

Various health organizations, including the Centers for Disease Control and Prevention (CDC) and the National Institutes of Health (NIH), officially define the terms *overweight* and *obesity* using the body mass index (BMI), which factors in a person's weight relative to height. Most of these organizations define an overweight adult as having a BMI between 25 and 29.9, while an obese adult is anyone who has a BMI of 30 or higher.[1] If you would like a chart to help you determine your BMI, refer to my book *The Seven Pillars of Health* or conduct an online search for "BMI" and take advantage of the many Web sites with tools to help you calculate your BMI.

However, I believe an even more important measurement to focus on is your waist size. The larger your waist, the greater your chances of having type 2 diabetes. In fact, it's been proven that, for men, waist size is an even better predictor of diabetes than BMI. A thirteen-year study of more than twenty-seven thousand men discovered that:

- A waist size of 34 to 36 doubled diabetes risk.

- A waist size of 36 to 38 nearly tripled the risk.

- A waist size of 38 to 40 was associated with five times the risk.

- A waist size of 40 to 62 was associated with twelve times the risk.[2]

DR. COLBERT'S RAPID WAIST REDUCTION DIET

This Bible cure combines faith in God with practical steps, as you know by now. So, here is the practical side: the diet. I recommend you use the rules of good nutrition for diabetics outlined in chapter 17 on nutrition and create a daily diet using my Rapid Waist Reduction Diet. The key is to eat no complex carbs after 6:00 p.m. other than beans or lentils. Make sure to choose the *organic* form of any of the allowable foods listed below.

Allowable foods

Breakfast

- Two to three free-range or organic eggs, omega-3 egg yolk, three egg whites per day, or one scoop of Life's Basics Plant Protein (see appendix) with 8 oz. of coconut milk, coconut kefir (from a health food store), skim milk, or low-fat plain kefir
- Two- to three-egg omelet with plenty of veggies (onions, avocado, tomatoes, etc.); use one whole egg or three egg whites
- ½ cup steel-cut oatmeal (tennis ball–sized serving) or the new high-fiber instant oatmeal (if time is a factor)
- 1 Tbsp. almonds, walnuts, or pecans
- ½ cup berries, one Granny Smith apple, or one pear

Lunch

- As much salad as you want. Salads may include any of the following: avocado, celery, chives, cilantro, cucumber, greens, parsley, red or yellow peppers, sprouts, and tomatoes.
- A sweet potato the size of a tennis ball, or ½ cup beans, peas, or lentils
- Homemade salad dressings in a salad spritzer (dressing can be made using four parts vinegar to one part extra-virgin olive oil and may include garlic, lime, lemon, and cilantro), or you may use salad spritzers such as Ken's or Wishbone
- 1 Tbsp. of seeds or nuts (1 Tbsp. = about ten nuts), or 1 Tbsp. of any of the following oils: grape seed oil mayonnaise, extra-virgin olive oil, coconut butter, organic butter (check labels to make sure you choose oils that are non GMO)
- Vegetable or bean soup (non-cream-based soups)
- 3–4 oz. for females or 4–5 oz. for males of lean protein (chicken, turkey, tongol tuna, salmon, sardines,

extra-lean red meat, etc.) grilled, baked, or broiled, not fried (limit red meat to 18 oz. or less a week)

Dinner

- 3–5 oz. of protein (allowable sources of protein are lean meats, poultry, eggs, and fish such as wild Alaskan salmon, tongol tuna, and sardines)

- As many steamed, stir-fried, grilled, or raw vegetables as you want. Allowable veggies are asparagus, bok choy, broccoli, brussels sprouts, cabbage, cauliflower, celery, chard, Chinese cabbage, eggplant, green beans, green chilies, kale, leeks, onions, snow peas, sprouts, tomatoes, and zucchini. Many foods from Thailand typically (or Thai restaurants) contain these veggies.

- Fresh herbs and spices to flavor foods to taste

- Salad and salad dressing, as described on the previous page

- ½ cup legumes and beans, peas, or lentils (tennis ball–sized serving); bean soup; or hummus

Beverages

- Lemonade or limeade made from fresh lemon or lime with water, sweetened with stevia

- Green, white, or black tea sweetened with stevia

Foods to limit or avoid

- Dairy: if you must eat dairy, eat it for breakfast, and limit it to skim or 1 percent organic milk or organic, plain, low-fat kefir and yogurt (I prefer coconut kefir)

- Grains, including flours made from grains (wheat, rice, barley, millet, rye, spelt, corn, popcorn)—except occasional steel-cut oatmeal for breakfast

- Pasta, bread, crackers, cookies, flour, and cereal

- French fries

- Fruit juice

- Pineapple, banana, grapes, raisins, and bottled or canned fruit or fruit juice
- Fast food and soft drinks
- Sweetened yogurt and kefir, whole and 2 percent milk and ice cream
- Glucose, dextrose, sucrose, corn syrup, honey, sugar, maple syrup, or maltodextrin
- Diet drinks and artificial sweeteners
- Hydrogenated vegetable oil, margarine, Crisco, commercial mayo, and salad dressing
- MSG (monosodium glutamate) in soups or any other foods
- Canola oil
- Peanuts and peanut food products

Treats and cheats (for weekends only; best to eat before 3:00 p.m.; commit to this program for thirty days before cheating)

- ½ cup of whole fruit (allowable fruits are grapefruit, whole oranges, kiwi, strawberries, cranberries, watermelon, raspberries, peaches, blueberries, blackberries, and apricots)
- ½ cup of certain whole grains (allowable whole grains are brown rice pasta, fiber crisp crackers, 100 percent buckwheat Japanese soba noodles, and organic brown rice)
- Potato (allowable potatoes are half of a baked potato with one pat of organic butter, half of a serving of mashed potatoes, and homemade french fries made from stir-frying potato wedges in coconut butter)
- Refried beans made with extra-virgin olive oil

SIMPLE RULES

The following are simple dieting rules that I always recommend to my patients who need to lose weight, especially belly fat:

1. Graze throughout the day. (Eat lots of salads and veggies often throughout the day.)

2. Eat a large breakfast. Eat breakfast like a king, lunch like a prince, and dinner like a pauper.

3. Eat smaller midmorning and midafternoon snacks, such as recommended protein bars and coconut milk kefir blended with Life's Basics Plant Protein.

4. Avoid all simple sugar foods such as candies, cookies, cakes, pies, and doughnuts. If you must have sugar, use either stevia, Sweet Balance, or Just Like Sugar (found in health food stores.)

5. Drink two quarts of filtered or bottled water a day. It is best to drink two 8-oz. glasses thirty minutes before each meal, or one to two 8-oz. glasses two and a half hours after each meal, and 8 to 16 oz. upon waking.

6. Avoid alcohol.

7. Avoid all fried foods.

8. Avoid, or decrease dramatically, starches. Starches include all breads, crackers, bagels, potatoes, pasta, rice, and corn. Limit beans to ½ cup one to two times a day. Also avoid bananas and dried fruit.

9. Eat fresh low-glycemic fruits only for breakfast or lunch; steamed, stir-fried, or raw vegetables; lean meats; salads (preferably with extra-virgin olive oil and vinegar); almonds and seeds.

10. Take fiber supplements such as one to three capsules of PGX fiber with 16 oz. of water before each meal. (See appendix B.)

11. For snacks, choose bars such as Jay Robb bars, gluten-free bars, and chocolate flaxseed bars. Try to limit these bars to one or two a day. These may be purchased at a health food store. Refer to *Dr. Colbert's "I Can Do This" Diet* for more information.

12. Do not eat past 7:00 p.m.

> For God has not given us a spirit of fear and timidity, but of power, love, and self-discipline.
>
> —2 TIMOTHY 1:7, NLT

I strongly recommend my book *Dr. Colbert's "I Can Do This" Diet* for weight loss. Start every day with prayer to God for success. Speak aloud the Bible verses that are scattered throughout this book. In addition, plan your menu each day, and follow these additional simple rules. With a little patience, you'll be well on your way to that slimmer person you pictured when you closed your eyes—the healthy person God intended you to be!

FAITH MOVES MOUNTAINS

Feel like you've got a mountain of extra weight to lose? Don't be discouraged. You did not gain it overnight, and losing it overnight would not be healthy. Jesus Christ taught that any mountain of bondage will move when faith is applied. Look at the verse: "'You don't have enough faith,' Jesus told them. 'I tell you the truth, if you had faith even as small as a mustard seed, you could say to this mountain, "Move from here to there," and it would move. Nothing would be impossible'" (Matt. 17:20, NLT).

Let me teach you something about faith. Faith is the most powerful force in the universe. Absolutely nothing is impossible to a person with faith. Faith is a belief that you already have what you are believing for. "[He] calls those things which do not exist as though they did" (Rom. 4:17, NKJV). Your daily vision and your daily confession then feed your faith. Your faith is similar to planting a seed, and the vision and confession are the seeds receiving nutrients—sunshine and water. On the other hand, getting discouraged and speaking defeat is similar to digging up your seed. Listen carefully: Faith is not a feeling or an emotion. It is a choice—a decision to believe God's Word despite everything else to the contrary. I have watched faith move many mountains. I have seen many people rise from wheelchairs and be healed by the power of the Holy Spirit. They were no different from you. They didn't think higher thoughts or come from more godly families. However, they did choose to believe God, to have a vision of themselves healed, and to make a daily confession of their healing. It's so simple.

Choose faith, and apply it right now to your situation.

A **BIBLE CURE** *Prayer for You*

Lord, I surrender the entire issue of weight control to You. Help me to face this issue in my life and find new hope, fresh vision, and powerful victory in You. Your Word says, "Nothing is impossible with God." I choose to believe Your Word right now and surrender and cast down all my feelings and thoughts of defeat in the arena of weight control. Thank You for loving me just as I am. And thank You for helping me to control my weight so that I will live a longer and better life. Amen.

A **BIBLE CURE** *Prescription*

Create a Sample Menu

Step 1: Start with prayer for success.

Step 2: Select a victory verse.

Step 3: Today's menu based upon the allowable foods from my Rapid Waist Reduction Diet:

Breakfast:

_____

_____

_____

Lunch:

_____

_____

_____

Dinner:

_____

_____

_____

Snacks:

_____

_____

_____

In addition, I will implement the following simple rules:

- Graze throughout the day. (Eat lots of salads and veggies often throughout the day.)

- Eat a large breakfast.

- Eat smaller midmorning and midafternoon snacks.

- Avoid all simple sugar foods such as candies, cookies, cakes, pies, and doughnuts.

- Drink two quarts of filtered or bottled water a day.

- Other:

Chapter 20

BATTLE DIABETES WITH NUTRIENTS AND SUPPLEMENTS

THERE ARE GOD-CREATED ways for you to add nutrients and supplements to your diet to begin controlling your blood sugar in a systematic, natural way. Both type 1 and type 2 diabetes can be helped by nutritional supplements. You must remember that supplements cannot take the place of a complete program to control and reverse type 2 diabetes that includes a focus on weight reduction, a good dietary plan, a regular exercise program, as well as stress reduction and hormone replacement therapy.

Following is a complete list of nutrients and supplements that will help you fight type 2 diabetes. (If you have type 1 diabetes, these supplements are still helpful to your overall health; however, the supplements listed below that will be of greatest benefit in fighting your form of diabetes are alpha lipoic acid, vitamin D, chromium, PGX fiber, omega-3, and the supplements for decreasing glycation.)

A good multivitamin

The foundation of a good supplement program always starts with a good comprehensive multivitamin. Adequate doses of nutrients found in a good multivitamin include magnesium, vanadium, biotin and the B vitamins, and the macro minerals and trace minerals.

- Magnesium is essential for glucose balance and is important for the release of insulin and the maintenance of the pancreatic beta cells, which produce insulin. Magnesium also increases the affinity and number of insulin receptors, which are on the surface of cells. The recommended daily allowance for magnesium is 350 mg a day for men and 280 mg a day for women.

- Vanadium is another mineral that assists in the metabolism of glucose.
- Biotin is a B vitamin that helps prevent insulin resistance.

Even though a multivitamin is extremely important in forming the foundation of a nutritional supplement program, there are other key nutrients or a larger dose of certain vitamins and minerals that you need to take in addition to a good comprehensive multivitamin. Most physicians are unaware of which nutritional supplements are effective in lowering blood sugar levels. You will need to make your physician aware that you are taking supplements for diabetes. The supplements alone are able to lower one's blood sugar significantly, and diabetic medication dosages will eventually need to be lowered accordingly. However, when the nutritional supplements are combined with weight loss, regular exercise, my dietary program, stress reduction, and hormone replacement, the results are typically profound.

Vitamin D

Many Americans are not getting enough vitamin D, and we are beginning to see a close link between vitamin D deficiency and diabetes. A recent article published by researchers from Loyola University's Marcella Niehoff School of Nursing concluded that an adequate intake of vitamin D may prevent or delay the onset of diabetes as well as decrease complications for those who are diagnosed with diabetes. This article substantiated the role of vitamin D in the prevention as well as management of glucose intolerance and diabetes.[1]

Vitamin D also plays an important role in the secretion of insulin and in helping you avoid insulin resistance. Vitamin D not only decreases your blood sugar but also increases your body's sensitivity to insulin, thus make insulin more effective.

I check vitamin D levels on most of my patients by checking the 25-OHD3 level. I typically try to get the patient's vitamin D level greater than fifty and less than one hundred. I typically start most of my patients on 2,000 IU of vitamin D a day and may increase that amount to 4,000 or even 6,000 IU a day as I continue to monitor their 25-OHD3 level until the vitamin D level is greater than fifty. I then place them on a maintenance dose of vitamin D.

Chromium

Chromium is a mineral that is essential for good health. It has been of interest to diabetes researchers for a long time because it is required for normal metabolism of sugar, carbs, protein, and fat. Chromium is like insulin's little helper, and without adequate chromium, insulin cannot function properly.

How much chromium do you need? In 1989, the National Academy of Sciences recommended an intake range for adults and adolescents of 50 to 200 mcg of chromium daily.[2] The Food and Nutrition Board of the Institute of Medicine has since narrowed this range down to 35 mcg for men and 25 mcg for women ages nineteen to fifty.[3]

A well-balanced diet should always be your first step in getting adequate amounts of vitamins, minerals, and other nutrients; however, fewer and fewer foods are providing the needed dietary intake levels of this important mineral. Whole grains and mushrooms may contain trace amounts of chromium, but that is only if these foods are grown in soils containing chromium. Likewise, seafood and some meat contain chromium, but only if the foods the animals ate contained chromium. Brewer's yeast is the only natural food source high in chromium; however, very few people eat this on a regular basis.

Also the standard American diet, full of refined sugars and carbohydrates, actually *depletes* your body of chromium since these foods require chromium for metabolism. I recommend you avoid foods high in refined sugars and carbs and consider taking chromium in supplement form.

Type 2 diabetics in particular tend to be deficient in chromium, whether as a cause or result of their condition. For this reason, I especially recommend supplementing chromium if you have type 2 diabetes.

A **BIBLE CURE** Health Fact

Selected Food Sources of Chromium[4]

A well-balanced diet does provide you with some chromium; however, the methods used for growing and manufacturing certain foods greatly affect their chromium levels and make it difficult to determine specific amounts of chromium you receive from each food. The following chart shows approximate chromium levels in foods, but it should only be used as a general guide.

Food	Chromium (mcg)
Broccoli, ½ cup	11
Grape juice, 1 cup	8
English muffin, whole wheat, 1	4
Potatoes, mashed, 1 cup	3
Garlic, dried, 1 teaspoon	3
Basil, dried, 1 tablespoon	2
Beef cubes, 3 ounces	2
Orange juice, 1 cup	2
Turkey breast, 3 ounces	2
Whole wheat bread, 2 slices	2
Red wine, 5 ounces	1–13
Apple, unpeeled, 1 medium	1
Banana, 1 medium	1
Green beans, ½ cup	1

Richard A. Anderson, PhD, chief chemist at the USDA Nutrient Requirements and Functions Laboratory, has conducted many studies on chromium supplementation and its effects on diabetes. He says, "Increased intake of chromium has been shown to lead to improvements in glucose, insulin, lipids, and related variables."[5]

Be aware that chromium is commonly included in multivitamins, usually in amounts ranging from 100 to 200 mcg. For many people this may provide adequate supplementation.[6] Always inform your doctor before making any changes to your diet or supplement program; however, realize that most doctors are unaware of this information.

There are several forms of chromium used for supplementation, but the most common form is chromium picolinate. For my type 2 diabetic patients, I typically recommend supplementing chromium picolinate in the amount of 600 to 1,000 mcg a day in divided doses.

One study conducted by Dr. Anderson found that type 2 diabetics who consumed 1,000 mcg per day of chromium improved insulin sensitivity without significant changes in body fat; type 1 diabetics were able to reduce their insulin dosage by 30 percent after only ten days of supplemental chromium picolinate at 200 mcg per day.[7]

Other studies in which researchers gave chromium to people with type 1 and type 2 diabetes have yielded mixed results. However, Dr. Anderson says that studies that show no beneficial effects using chromium for diabetes were usually using doses of chromium of 200 mcg or less, which is simply inadequate for diabetes, especially if the chromium is in the form that is poorly absorbed.[8]

Can you take too much chromium? According to Dr. Anderson's research, no discernible toxicity has been found in rats that consumed levels up to several thousand times the dietary reference for chromium for humans (based on body weight). There have also been no documented toxic effects in any of the human studies involving supplemental chromium, according to Dr. Anderson.[9] But again, please don't take massive amounts of any supplement without the advice of your doctor.

Alpha lipoic acid

Alpha lipoic acid is an important nutrient for fighting both type 1 and type 2 diabetes. Diabetics are more prone to oxidative stress and free radical formation than nondiabetics. Lipoic acid is an amazing antioxidant that works in both water-soluble and fat-soluble compartments of the body and regenerates vitamin C, vitamin E, coenzyme Q_{10}, and glutathione. Lipoic acid also improves insulin resistance in overweight adults suffering from type 2 diabetes.

Lipoic acid can also help relieve several components of metabolic syndrome: it can lower blood pressure, decrease insulin resistance, improve the lipid profile, and help individuals lose weight. Lipoic acid has also been used in Europe for decades to treat diabetic neuropathy with amazing success.

I usually start my diabetic patients on 300 mg of alpha lipoic acid twice a day, monitoring their blood sugars, and I may occasionally go up to 300 mg three times a day. Some patients develop GI side effects, skin allergies, or decreased thyroid function, so I monitor these tests closely while a patient is taking lipoic acid. Scientific studies using doses ranging from 300 mg to 1,800 mg a day infer that the most important form of lipoic acid is R-dihydro-lipoic acid, which is the most readily available form.[10] However, I find that alpha lipoic acid usually works best for the diabetic patients I have treated.

Cinnamon

The Chinese have used cinnamon medicinally for over four thousand years. Ancient Egyptians and Romans also recognized its many uses, and it has remained one of the most common spices in the world to this day.

In recent years, cinnamon's therapeutic effects have made headlines as some research has shown that cinnamon may have an insulin-like effect and cause blood sugar to be stored in the form of glycogen. It also contains excellent antioxidant properties.

The most commonly cited study on the effects of cinnamon in diabetes was published in *Diabetes Care* in 2003. Sixty people with type 2 diabetes were divided into six groups of ten patients each. Groups one through three were treated with 1, 3, or 6 g of cinnamon per day, and groups four through six received a placebo. After forty days, the cinnamon group's reduction in blood sugar was amazing. Their fasting blood sugars were lowered by 18 to 29 percent. The placebo group, however, showed no change.[11]

Whole cinnamon contains oils that may trigger allergic reactions. This is why I recommend a cinnamon extract instead. One form of cinnamon extract is Cinnulin PF, which contains the active component found in whole cinnamon without the toxins. USDA studies have indicated that cinnamon extract promotes glucose metabolism and healthy cholesterol levels in people with type 2 diabetes.[12] Cinnamon extract also appears to help glucose transport mechanisms by increasing the insulin signaling pathways. I generally recommend taking 250 mg of Cinnulin PF twice a day.

Soluble fiber

As I mentioned in chapter 17, soluble fiber not only helps to slow the digestion of starches, but it also slows glucose uptake and thus lowers the glycemic index of your meal. This in turn lowers the amount of insulin that is secreted by the pancreas, which is very beneficial for those with type 2 diabetes. Soluble fiber has also been shown over the years through numerous studies to effectively lower blood sugar levels.[13]

How does it do all of these things? Soluble fiber actually swells many times its original size as it binds to the water in your stomach and small intestine to form a gluelike gel that not only slows down the absorption of glucose but also induces a sense of satiety (fullness) and reduces your body's absorption of calories.

High-fiber diets

Studies conducted by James W. Anderson, MD, of the University of Kentucky, showed that high-fiber diets lowered insulin requirements an average of 38 percent in people with type 1 diabetes and 97 percent in people with type 2 diabetes. This means that almost all of the people suffering from type 2 diabetes who followed Dr. Anderson's high-fiber diet were able to lower or stop taking insulin and other diabetes medications and still maintain a healthy blood sugar level. Additionally, these results lasted up to fifteen years.[14]

Fruit, beans, chickpeas, lentils, carrots, squash, oat bran, barley, rice bran, guar gum, glucomannan, and pectin are all very good sources of soluble fiber.

Supplementing with PGX

Of course, in addition to dietary sources of fiber, it's a good idea to supplement. I recommend a specific fiber supplement developed by scientists at the University of Toronto called PGX (short for PolyGlycopleX). Often called the new "super fiber," PGX is a unique blend of plant fibers containing glucomannan, a soluble and fermentable fiber derived from the root of the konjac plant. It also contains sodium alginate, xanthan gum, and mulberry leaf extract. It works the same as dietary sources of fiber; however, the specific ratio of natural compounds used in PGX enable it to be three to five times as effective as other fibers alone.

Clinical studies by Dr. Vuksan, the developer of PGX, have shown repeatedly that blood sugar levels after meals decrease as soluble fiber viscosity increases.[15] The exciting news is that PGX fiber lowers after-meal blood sugars by approximately 20 percent and also lowers insulin secretion by approximately 40 percent. This is unequaled by any drug or natural health-food product.

Recently, researchers at the University of Toronto found that higher doses of PGX can decrease appetite significantly because PGX absorbs six hundred times its weight in water over one to two hours and expands in the digestive tract.[16]

Most soluble fiber has side effects of producing significant amounts of gas; however, PGX has fewer GI side effects than other dietary fiber, mainly because PGX can be given in much smaller quantities than other viscous fibers and achieve comparable health benefits without all the gas.[17]

Any time you increase your fiber intake, you should start slowly and drink plenty of water. With PGX, I recommend that you start with one capsule, three times a day before meals, with 16 oz. of water, and gradually increase the dose as tolerated every two to three days. Most people use two to three softgels before meals with 16 oz. of water. Rarely will someone need six softgels before meals, which is the maximum dose.

Irvingia

Irvingia is a fruit-bearing plant from the jungles of Cameroon. It is believed that Irvingia has the ability to enable one to lose weight by simply lowering CRP (C-reactive protein) levels, which in turn lowers leptin resistance.[18]

Leptin is a hormone that tells your brain you've eaten enough and it's time to stop. It also enhances your body's ability to use fat as an energy source.

Unfortunately, because of sedentary lifestyles and the many highly processed, high-glycemic food choices available through the standard American diet, many overweight and obese patients have acquired resistance to leptin, and this hormone no longer works properly in their bodies. Similar to insulin resistance, leptin resistance is a chronic inflammatory condition that contributes to weight gain as well as belly fat.

This is why the new research demonstrating Irvingia's promise in reversing leptin resistance is so important. In one double-blind study, 102 overweight volunteers took either 150 mg of Irvingia or a placebo twice a day for ten weeks. At the end of ten weeks, the Irvingia group lost on average of 28 pounds with 6.7 inches lost from their waistlines. The Irvingia group also had a 32 percent reduction in fasting blood sugar, 26 percent reduction in total cholesterol, and 52 percent reduction in CRP.[19]

I have been using Irvingia with my diabetic patients since 2008 and have seen remarkable improvements in most of their blood sugar measurements as well their hemoglobin A1C levels. The dose that is generally recommended is 150 mg of standardized Irvingia extract two times a day.

Omega-3 fatty acids

Omega-3 fats are simply polyunsaturated fats that come from foods such as fish, fish oil, vegetable oils (especially flaxseed oil), walnuts, and wheat germ. However, the most beneficial omega-3 fats are fish oils containing EPA and DHA.

Omega-3 fats generally protect against heart disease, decrease inflammation, lower triglyceride levels, and may help prevent insulin resistance and improve glucose tolerance. Fish oil also helps to decrease the rate of developing diabetic vascular complications. Omega-3 fats also decrease inflammation, help to reduce the risk of heart disease and stroke, and slow the progression of atherosclerosis.

Even though fish oils are probably the most protective fats for our blood vessels, trans fats are actually the worst fats for our blood vessels and also can greatly increase one's risk of developing diabetes. Trans fats are hydrogenated fats or partially hydrogenated fats and are ubiquitous in both processed and fast food as well as served in many restaurants and restaurant chains. A recent study showed that only a 2 percent increase in calories from trans fat raised the risk of diabetes in females by 39 percent, and a 5 percent increase in polyunsaturated fats decreased the risk of diabetes by 37 percent.[20]

Dietary fats that are considered to be beneficial include not only fish oils but also avocados, extra-virgin olive oil, almond butter, nuts, and seeds.

A word of caution since some fish oil supplements may contain mercury, pesticides, or PCBs. See appendix B for fish oil (omega-3) products I recommend as safe.

I usually place my patients with prediabetes and those with diabetes on 320 to 1,000 mg of fish oils three times a day. If they have high triglyceride levels, I may increase the dose to 4,000 to 5,000 mg a day.

SUPPLEMENTS TO DECREASE GLYCATION

Carnosine

Glycation is the name for protein molecules that bind to glucose molecules and form advanced glycation end products (AGEs). Glycated proteins produce fifty times more free radicals than nonglycated proteins. Typical manifestations of this are skin wrinkling and brain degeneration. Both prediabetics and diabetics are much more prone to glycation and, as a result, will age prematurely.

The amino acid carnosine, however, helps stabilize and protect cell membranes from glycation. Carnosine is a safe and effective nutrient for inhibiting glycation. I usually recommend at least 1,000 mg a day of carnosine to my diabetic patients.

Pyridoxamine

A unique form of vitamin B_6 called pyridoxamine interferes with accelerated glycation reactions in diabetics. Glycation end products are closely linked with diabetic kidney disease, diabetic retinopathy, and diabetic neuropathy. However, pyridoxamine is one of the most powerful natural supplements for inhibiting AGE formation and has been found to be superior to the other two forms of vitamin B_6 in inhibiting AGE formation and glycation.

> Do not carouse with drunkards or feast with gluttons, for they are on their way to poverty, and too much sleep clothes them in rags.
> —PROVERBS 23:20–21, NLT

Pyridoxamine has been studied clinically in the treatment of diabetic kidney disease. Trials at the Joslin Diabetes Center at Harvard

Medical School are promising using pyridoxamine and suggest a protective effect of kidney function in diabetics.[21]

Neurological problems can occur when you consume megadoses (more than 2,000 mg per day); therefore, I recommend you stay on the safe side with a dose of 50 mg (one capsule) of pyridoxamine, taken with food once a day.

Benfotiamine

Benfotiamine is a fat-soluble form of vitamin B_1 and has been shown to help prevent the development as well as progression of many diabetic complications. This has been used in Europe for decades as a prescription medication. It helps to slow the progression of diabetic nerve, kidney, and retinal disease, and also helps to relieve diabetic neuropathy. Benfotiamine is fat soluble, so it can easily enter cells and help prevent dysfunction associated with diabetes within the cells.

A recent double-blind study in Germany found that diabetic patients with polyneuropathy who were given 100 mg of benfotiamine four times a day for three weeks had statistically significant improvement in nerve function scores.[22]

Benfotiamine offers protection for the nerves, kidneys, retina, and vascular system from damage caused by diabetes. That is why supplementation is extremely important in preventing long-term complications of type 1 and type 2 diabetes. My recommended dose is 100 mg four times a day.

A **BIBLE CURE** Health Tip

Dr. Colbert's Diabetic Protocol

I place all of my diabetic patients on a comprehensive multivitamin, as well as omega-3 fat. I also typically place them on vitamin D, chromium, alpha lipoic acid, cinnulin, Irvingia, and PGX fiber. I generally will add a supplement to prevent glycation such as carnosine, pyridoxamine, or benfotiamine. I usually start pyridoxamine if they are developing symptoms of glycation, such as kidney disease, neuropathy, or retinopathy. For more information on supplements as well as more in-depth dietary and exercise information, please refer to my book *The Seven Pillars of Health*.

SUPPLEMENTS TO REPLENISH HORMONES

Balancing hormones is extremely important in managing diabetes. Elevated stress hormone levels are associated with increased belly fat and increased insulin resistance, causing decreased blood sugar control. Sex hormone deficiency has actually decreased the effectiveness of insulin. It is interesting to note that aging is associated with a decrease in sex hormone levels and an increase in the incidence of type 2 diabetes.

Testosterone

Testosterone is the male hormone that is associated with increased muscle mass, deepening of the voice, and male pattern hair growth. High testosterone levels are associated with a significantly lower risk of type 2 diabetes in men. On the other hand, low levels of testosterone in males have repeatedly been shown to be associated with an increased risk of type 2 diabetes as well as abdominal obesity.

> Let all that I am praise the LORD; with my whole heart, I will praise his holy name. Let all that I am praise the LORD; may I never forget the good things he does for me. He forgives all my sins and heals all my diseases.
>
> —PSALM 103:1–3, NLT

Testosterone replacement therapy decreases insulin resistance and improves blood sugar control in men with low testosterone levels. In all men with type 2 diabetes, I always check both total and free testosterone levels, and I have found that a large percentage of men with type 2 diabetes indeed have low testosterone levels. I then typically place them on a small amount of transdermal testosterone cream in order to raise their testosterone levels to normal. To find a doctor knowledgeable in hormone replacement therapy (HRT), please see appendix B.

It is interesting to note that high testosterone levels are also associated with a higher risk of type 2 diabetes in females. I believe the reason for this is that many women with high testosterone levels also have large waist measurements or increased belly fat.

Also, women with high testosterone levels may have polycystic ovary syndrome (PCOS). PCOS runs in families and is associated with insulin resistance; infertility; increased hair on the face, arms, and legs; acne; obesity; and elevated testosterone levels. They are also at a significant increased risk of developing type 2 diabetes.

PCOS gets its name from early cases that were associated with multiple cysts of the ovaries. However, this is not a main feature of this condition even though the name has stuck.

It is also interesting to note that PCOS can be managed with a very low glycemic diet as well as exercise. Many physicians also use the diabetic medication metformin, which helps control the blood sugar.

A **BIBLE CURE** *Health Tip*

Medications for Polycystic Ovary Syndrome[23]

Because there is no cure for PCOS, it needs to be managed very carefully. Most physicians prescribe a combination of treatments based on their specific symptoms. These treatments include birth control pills, diabetes medications, antiandrogens to decrease the impact of male hormones, and even surgery.

Research shows that more than 50 percent of women with PCOS are likely to have prediabetes or diabetes before the age of forty. Keeping the symptoms of PCOS under control is the best way to reduce your risk of developing complications like diabetes, heart disease, and cancer. Regular testing for diabetes, eating right, exercising, and not smoking are also very helpful in reducing your chances of developing serious health problems associated with PCOS. Also, the supplements for type 2 diabetes will also help PCOS, but diet and regular exercise are absolutely critical for managing it.

Estrogen

It is interesting to note that when many women go through menopause, they typically develop a *menopot*, or potbelly, as well as increased truncal obesity. As their weight gradually increases, their cholesterol typically increases, their blood pressure usually rises, and their blood sugar level also typically rises.

If you are a woman, a very important function of estrogen is that it fights insulin resistance by improving the effectiveness of insulin, helping to lower your blood sugar. Estrogen also helps redistribute the fat from your waist to your hips, buttocks, and thigh areas. Estrogen increases your metabolic rate and helps you maintain muscle mass as well.

In other words, estrogen helps prevent diabetes. But unfortunately, most doctors do not prescribe transdermal bioidentical estrogen but synthetic estrogen in pill form, such as Premarin (a prescription estrogen medication made from pregnant mare's urine), which causes more weight gain and a greater risk of diabetes. Premarin is the most common prescribed estrogen and is associated with weight gain. I've helped so many women over the years control their blood sugar and lose weight by balancing their hormones with bioidentical transdermal hormone creams. To find a doctor knowledgeable in HRT in your area, please refer to appendix B.

Progesterone

In women, it is also critically important to balance estrogen with progesterone, the other female hormone. Progesterone actually helps to balance estrogen levels. Progesterone also has a natural calming effect on the body and helps one to sleep. This helps to lower cortisol levels, which will also help lower blood sugar levels.

However, most women are taking synthetic progesterone, such as Provera, or taking large doses of bioidentical progesterone. When women take either synthetic progesterone or too much natural progesterone, it decreases glucose tolerance or may predispose one to developing diabetes. Progesterone can also increase insulin and cortisol levels, setting you up for increased belly fat and rising blood sugar levels.

Now, hopefully you are beginning to understand the importance of balancing these very important hormones and checking the levels of these hormones.

Wise words satisfy like a good meal; the right words bring satisfaction. The tongue can bring death or life; those who love to talk will reap the consequences.

—PROVERBS 18:20–21, NLT

A FINAL NOTE

As you have observed, there are many nutrients and supplements that can help you effectively battle diabetes. If you are a type 2 diabetic and you choose to follow this program and monitor your blood sugar, you should find that your blood sugar is likely to drop within the normal range in a few months.

If you are a type 1 diabetic, until you receive complete divine healing from God, you will always be on insulin. However, you may be able to lower your dosage of insulin by following the measures outlined in this book.

Regularly consult with your physician, and use these vitamins and nutrients as he or she may recommend. God has created these wonderful natural substances to empower us in maintaining good health and overcoming the debilitating effects of diabetes.

A **BIBLE CURE** *Prayer for You*

Heavenly Father, help me apply these things I have learned in my battle against diabetes. Help me eat wisely and obtain my ideal body weight. Show me which vitamins, minerals, and supplements will best help my body fight diabetes. Heal my body so that insulin will be produced and then used by my cells in a healthy way. Strengthen my resolve to exercise regularly. Keep me in Your divine health so that I may live a long, productive life serving You. Amen.

A **BIBLE CURE** *Prescription*

Winning the Battle Over Diabetes

List the vitamins, minerals, and supplements you now take.

_____

_____

_____

_____

_____

_____

What supplements do you plan to add in order to treat diabetes?

_____

_____

_____

_____

_____

If you are a male, have you had your total and free testosterone levels checked? If you are a female and are menopausal or premenopausal, have you had your hormone levels checked? Are you taking synthetic estrogen or synthetic progesterone in pill form? If so, see a doctor knowledgeable in bioidentical hormones.

_____

_____

_____

_____

Chapter 21

BATTLE DIABETES WITH SPIRITUAL AND EMOTIONAL STRENGTH

HAVE YOU BEEN told that you have diabetes? As a Christian physician, I can tell you that you do need to believe God for a miracle. Balanced with that, it is necessary for you to do your part to take care of your health. But if miracles happened every time we wanted them to happen, they wouldn't be miracles anymore—they would be cures!

Miracles are a divine touch, a moment of supernatural intervention when total healing occurs—but all healing is from God. A doctor can sew up an incision and bind up a wound. But the power that heals the wound and makes you well again always comes from God. I encourage you to pray for a miracle, but don't stop there. Lay hold of the principles of health outlined in this book to aid the healing process. In addition, let's look at diabetes in another way that you may not have thought of.

ANOTHER DIMENSION

Throughout this book we have taken a close look at the physical side of diabetes. But another dimension exists to this disease that we must also address: a spiritual and emotional dimension.

> A merry heart does good, like medicine, but a broken spirit dries the bones.
>
> —PROVERBS 17:22, NKJV

The Bible strongly suggests that our health sometimes has an emotional and spiritual component. Do you know that negative emotions can affect your physical body? According to the Bible, they can.

LESS STRESS

One significant factor that will elevate your insulin level and make you vulnerable to diabetes is stress. As I discuss in my book *Stress Less*, it is common for people under chronic stress to have elevated levels of cortisol and insulin. At normal levels, cortisol (your body's stress hormone) counterbalances the effects of insulin. However, elevated cortisol decreases your sensitivity to insulin, which leads to insulin resistance.

In addition, elevated cortisol levels stimulate your appetite, producing a craving for sugars and carbohydrates—the very foods that keep your insulin levels elevated. By creating this vicious cycle, you can see how living with chronic stress programs your body for fat storage and obesity, and unfortunately, metabolic syndrome, prediabetes, and type 2 diabetes often follow.

God's plan is for you to handle stress by casting your cares on Him. "Give all your worries and cares to God, for he cares about you" (1 Pet. 5:7, NLT).

What cares have you neglected to give to God?

- Financial concerns
- Hurting relationships
- Future goals
- Job-related anxieties
- Other: _____

God cares for you and wants to see you through all the stress and worry you may be facing. If you hold on to your stress, then your body will suffer. Surrender your cares to Him.

TAKE THESE BIBLE CURE STEPS

I discuss the following stress busters in greater detail in my books *Stress Less* and *The Seven Pillars of Health*. But as I close this Bible Cure book, I'd like to briefly suggest the following steps to eliminate as much stress as possible from your life and greatly reduce the risks and complications of diabetes.

Enjoy the present moment.

This concept, often called "mindfulness," is the practice of learning to pay attention to what is happening to you from moment to moment. The definition of mindfulness reminds me of the words of Jesus:

> Therefore do not worry about tomorrow, for tomorrow will worry about its own things. Sufficient for the day is its own trouble.
>
> —MATTHEW 6:34, NKJV

Replace stress and worry about the future (or the past) with something to enjoy in the present moment.

Reframe your thinking.

While mindfulness is learning to live in the present moment, reframing is learning to see the past, present, and future in a positive light. When negative beliefs or thoughts pop up, challenge and assess them rather than automatically accepting them. This is what the apostle Paul meant when he said:

> Casting down imaginations, and every high thing that exalteth itself against the knowledge of God, and bringing into captivity every thought to the obedience of Christ.
>
> —2 CORINTHIANS 10:5, KJV

This is simply replacing your fears, worries, failures, grief, sorrows, and shame with God's promises. Reframing your thoughts in this way will lower your stress level and have a very real effect on your body.

Build margin into your life.

A very practical way to de-stress your life is to build margin into everything you do. Margin is a buffer between feeling overwhelmed and feeling at peace. Allowing yourself two hours to get to the airport when you only need one hour is margin. When you make a budget and only spend 80 percent of what you earn, that's margin.

Margin will not automatically appear in your schedule or finances. You must plan it and put it there. Learn to cut back on commitments, manage your time better, make a to-do list every night for the following day, build in time between appointments, spend less than you earn, pay off credit cards, and build up an emergency fund. These things will all build margin into your life, and your stress level will go down dramatically.

Remove obvious stressors, and surround yourself with positive people.

If you are under stress, it's likely that your environment includes stressors that can be removed. These might include clutter, an overcrowded schedule, or your relationships. Restoring order to your home or work environment is a proven stress reducer and slams the door on stress.

Now, I realize you can't completely avoid negative people or relationships, but I strongly encourage you to limit the amount of time you spend with them. Attitudes are contagious. Don't let their negative attitude drain all of your energy, joy, and strength. Instead, surround yourself with positive friends whose attitudes and words are those of love, thankfulness, appreciation, and humility.

Learn the power of "no."

Learning to say no is hard for some people, but it is very important. When you protect your time and energy because you realize how infinitely valuable they are to your mind, body, and spirit, you will avoid the stress that comes from overcommitting yourself and taking on problems or goals that are not your own. Instead, learn to assertively stand behind your own visions and goals for your life. Create healthy boundaries, and enforce them. You will find that your confidence increases as you do this, and your stress level will drop.

Pray.

Prayer is an unlimited resource for filling your life with God's Spirit, wisdom, strength, and peace. Philippians 4:6–7 says, "Be anxious for nothing, but in everything by prayer and supplication with thanksgiving let your requests be made known to God. And the peace of God, which surpasses all comprehension, will guard your hearts and your minds in Christ Jesus" (NASB).

Meditate on God's Word.

Throughout this book are scriptures that will strengthen and encourage you. Learn them. Speak them aloud. Let His Word bring guidance and healing into your life.

> But his delight is in the law of the LORD, and in His law he meditates day and night. He shall be like a tree planted by the rivers of water, that brings forth its fruit in its season, whose leaf also shall not wither; and whatever he does shall prosper.
>
> —PSALM 1:2–3, NKJV

A **BIBLE CURE** *Prayer for You*

Heavenly Father, help me to apply all of these things I have learned. I take Your hand for the rest of my journey through the seasons of my life. Help me to walk in divine health throughout the path You lay before me and to know You better all along the way. Lord, help me to speak and think positive words so that my life will bring help and refreshing to others. Give me the power to stop destructive habits and attitudes. Fill me with Your joy for life, and give me energy to take the necessary steps to stay fit, both physically and spiritually all of my days. Amen.

A **BIBLE CURE** *Prescription*

What cares have you neglected to give to God, resulting in stress in your life?

❏ Financial concerns
❏ Hurting relationships
❏ Future goals
❏ Job-related anxieties
❏ Other: _____

Check the spiritual steps you have started in overcoming diabetes:

❏ I am enjoying the present moment.
❏ I am reframing my thoughts.
❏ I am building margin into my life.
❏ I am eliminating obvious stressors.
❏ I am surrounding myself with positive people.
❏ I am learning to say no.
❏ I am praying.
❏ I am learning and applying God's Word.
❏ I am trusting God for health and strength.

Write a prayer thanking God for all the ways He has created to help you overcome diabetes in your life:

_____

_____

_____

_____

_____

_____

_____

_____

_____

THE BIBLE CURE

FOR CANDIDA & YEAST INFECTIONS

Chapter 22

YOU CAN RECLAIM YOUR HEALTH

Perhaps you've picked up this book wondering just what a Bible cure is all about. Maybe you've never before considered that God genuinely cares for your health. This Bible verse explains how He feels about your sicknesses.

"Jesus traveled through all the towns and villages of that area, teaching in the synagogues and announcing the Good News about the Kingdom. And he healed every kind of disease and illness. When he saw the crowds, he had compassion on them because they were confused and helpless, like sheep without a shepherd" (Matt. 9:35–36, NLT).

Not only does He care, but He also has great power to defeat all disease and sickness. God is greater than any disease or sickness that you will ever experience. The Bible says this about Jesus Christ: "For this reason also, God highly exalted Him, and bestowed on Him the name which is above every name, so that at the name of Jesus every knee will bow, of those who are in heaven and on earth and under the earth" (Phil. 2:9–10, NASB).

This verse simply says that Jesus Christ is higher and bigger than anything you will ever encounter. He is greater than all sickness and every disease. Because of that, every sickness and disease—no matter how great or small—must bow. That is the secret of His healing power.

You may have never before considered a Bible cure as an option in dealing with candida or yeast. If not, then get ready to reclaim your health in an entirely new way!

CANDIDA,
CANDIDIASIS AND YEAST INFECTIONS

Candida, candidiasis or the yeast syndrome is simply an overgrowth of yeast, usually in the intestinal tract and other tissues of the body. In women, painful yeast infections that infect the vagina can cause PMS and reduced sex drive.

Yeast can also overgrow in the GI tract, causing heartburn, indigestion, abdominal bloating, cramps, constipation or diarrhea, nausea and gas. Excessive yeast overgrowth is also related to environmental sensitivities and illnesses that heighten sensitivities to foods, chemicals such as smoke, chemical odors from carpets and fabrics and auto exhaust.

Yeast is everywhere. It's found in the food we eat and in the air we breathe, so it's impossible to avoid exposure to it. As a matter of fact, yeast normally lives in the human body. It flourishes in the warm, moist environment of the GI and vaginal tracts.

Still, you don't have to suffer from painful yeast attacks and overgrowth. There's a better way.

A BOLD, NEW APPROACH

With the help of the practical and faith-inspiring wisdom contained in this Bible Cure book, combined with alternative healing methods, you can beat yeast infections naturally.

Through the power of good nutrition, healthy lifestyle choices, exercise, vitamins and supplements, and most importantly of all, through the power of dynamic faith, you can halt the painful symptoms of debilitating yeast imbalances.

Enduring the pain and discomfort of candida and yeast syndrome is not God's will for you. With God's grace, perfect health and increasing joy await you!

So, as you read this book, prepare to triumph in your battle against candidiasis and yeast syndrome. This Bible Cure book is filled with practical steps, hope, encouragement and valuable information on how to develop a healthy, empowered lifestyle. In this book, you will

uncover God's divine plan of health for body, soul and
spirit through modern medicine, good nutrition and
the medicinal power of Scripture and prayer.

You will also discover life-changing scriptures throughout that will strengthen and encourage you.

As you read, apply and trust God's promises, you will also uncover powerful Bible Cure prayers to help you line up your thoughts and feelings with God's plan of divine health for you—a plan that includes living victoriously. You will find powerful insight in topics such as restoring your health with nutrition, renewing your body with supplements, recovering your edge with lifestyle changes, and recharging your spirit with faith.

You can confidently take the natural and spiritual steps outlined in this book to defeat candidiasis and yeast syndrome forever.

It is my prayer that these practical suggestions for health, nutrition and fitness will bring wholeness to your life—body, soul and spirit. May they deepen your fellowship with God and strengthen your ability to worship and serve Him.

A **BIBLE CURE** Prayer for You

Lord, You have revealed the causes for yeast syndrome, and in You are the remedies, cures and methods of prevention. Guide and direct me in applying this Bible cure method. Consecrate me, body, mind and spirit, to walk in divine health. Amen.

Chapter 23

GET INFORMED

W HETHER YOU REALIZE it or not, becoming better informed is actually a godly principle. The Bible says, "For the LORD grants wisdom! From his mouth come knowledge and understanding. He grants a treasure of common sense to the honest" (Prov. 2:6–7, NLT).

Wouldn't you like for God to grant you a treasure of good sense regarding your health? Of course you would! Getting God's wisdom and good sense begins with becoming better informed. In this chapter we will take a good look at candidiasis and yeast infections and develop a better understanding of the various causes for this painful problem and what can be done naturally to cure it.

CANDIDIASIS, A CLOSER LOOK

Yeast is actually a single-celled organism found everywhere: in water, air and on land. Candida is also present in all people from the first few months of life and usually lives harmoniously with us. What's destructive about yeast is how it can change from a harmless form to a dangerous invader.

When it changes forms, candida overgrowth can affect nearly every organ in the body and particularly the GI tract, nervous system, genital/urinary tract, endocrine system and immune system.

Under normal conditions yeast lives in our bodies without causing us any problems. Nearly three pounds of friendly bacteria in our intestines help to keep it in check. These friendly bacteria help our bodies maintain a balance of power between the good bacteria and the yeast.

That's until we upset this delicate balance with antibiotics, prednisone, hormones such as estrogen and progesterone, too much stress, diabetes or by eating too much sugar and highly processed foods. These things can swing the balance of power, causing an overgrowth of yeast to occur.

If this happens when your immune system is weakened, the harmless yeast can transform itself into an invasive fungal form.

> Then David asked the LORD, "Should I chase after this band of raiders? Will I catch them?" And the LORD told him, "Yes, go after them. You will surely recover everything that was taken from you!"
>
> —1 SAMUEL 30:8, NLT

This invasive form, called "mycelial form," actually produces rootlike tentacles called "rhizoids." These roots can then penetrate through the lining of the GI tract, causing a painful condition known as "leaky gut," which is increased intestinal permeability. When you have a leaky gut, partially digested food particles are able to pass through the intestinal lining and directly enter the bloodstream. Not only that, but toxic waste produced by the candida passes right into the bloodstream, too. When this happens, food allergies can result, as well as symptoms of excessive bloating, gas, belching, heartburn, diarrhea and constipation.

WHAT ARE THE SYMPTOMS?

Yeast produces more than seventy-nine known toxins. But probably the worst toxic substance produced by yeast is acetaldehyde. When this substance enters into the liver, it is then converted into alcohol. Acetaldehyde contributes to a raft of harmful symptoms. Here are a few of them:

- Fatigue
- Mental cloudiness
- Disorientation
- Confusion

- Irritability
- Headaches
- Anxiety
- Depression

Not only does yeast produce these distressing symptoms, but it also depletes minerals, increases free radical formation and disrupts enzymes needed to produce energy.

So you can see that yeast can invade the body, wreaking havoc wherever it goes. It also produces many different toxins that can make you feel absolutely miserable.

If yeast is given enough time, it can invade the bloodstream and may affect any organ or tissue in the entire body. As soon as a particular organ in your body is affected, symptoms begin to occur. For instance, as candida or its toxic waste products affect the nervous system, you may begin to experience the following symptoms:

- Fatigue
- Memory loss
- Insomnia
- Hyperactivity
- Autistic tendencies

- Sleepiness
- Attention-deficit disorder
- Depression
- Mood swings

AN AVALANCHE OF PHYSICAL COMPLAINTS

Left unchecked, candida overgrowth can sweep through your entire body like an avalanche. Before long every organ system can be affected. If your body is under a yeast attack, you may feel extremely fatigued much of the time. That's because yeast will often affect the endocrine system, eventually causing adrenal exhaustion and chronic fatigue. Thyroid problems can also be related to yeast overgrowth, including both overactive and underactive thyroid function. Skin problems such as eczema, hives, psoriasis and acne can develop, too.

As your body struggles to fight off the ravages of yeast overgrowth, eventually your immune system can be compromised. Food allergies may begin to surface as well as other food sensitivities.

Once candida weakens the digestive system, it becomes increasingly difficult to break down proteins into amino acids. When the partially digested proteins, called peptides, are absorbed directly into the bloodstream, your immune system recognizes them as foreign invaders. At this point your body may begin to form antibodies to attack them.

Often this immune reaction takes place in the lining of the small intestine, which therefore causes even more damage to the small intestines, leading to increased intestinal permeability, or leaky gut. A vicious cycle of destruction and allergic reactions spiral out of control.

Candida overgrowth in the small intestines can rob your body of vital nutrients. The toxic poisons that are excreted can poison your body's tissues.

What Causes Candida?

The most common reason that yeast grows out of control is due to excessive use of antibiotics. Many people have recurrent sinus infections, recurrent bladder infections, recurrent bouts of bronchitis or strep throat or prostatitis.

Many teenagers have severe acne and are on antibiotics such as tetracycline for years. Many times the acne is actually the result of candida. So, the acne may actually worsen rather than improve on tetracycline.

Because these people have repeatedly used antibiotics or have been on long-term antibiotics, these drugs eventually kill the majority of the good bacteria that live in the GI tract. Since the antibiotics do not affect candida, they multiply rapidly and may proliferate out of control. The yeast are normally held in check by the friendly bacteria, which have been killed by the antibiotics.

Antibiotics and Our Meat Supply

In addition, people who eat large amounts of beef, pork, chicken and veal will usually absorb small amounts of antibiotics and hormone residues. In 1991, the Centers for Disease Control in Atlanta revealed that half of the fifteen million pounds of antibiotics produced in America each year are used on livestock and poultry.[1] Many of the cattle, pigs and poultry have antibiotics added to their food routinely. As a result, residues of these antibiotics remain in many of the meats we eat.

Long-term antibiotics taken for chronic infections or consumed by eating large amounts of meat will eventually affect the delicate balance of good bacteria in the GI tract, leading to death of the good bacteria and an overgrowth of yeast.

Also, successive use of antibiotics is causing the development of resistant strains of bacteria. Antibiotic resistance is much more common when antibiotics are used frequently. If this trend continues, many infectious diseases may be almost impossible to treat due to antibiotic resistance.

SIDE EFFECTS FROM THE PILL

Birth control pills and the hormone progesterone are factors in developing candida overgrowth. When progesterone levels are high, such as during the second half of the menstrual cycle or during pregnancy, women are much more prone to develop yeast vaginitis. Corticosteroids such as prednisone are commonly associated with yeast overgrowth.

DO YOU HAVE CANDIDA?

We know that everyone has candida. Yes, it is actually present in all our GI tracts. But is the yeast in your body in balance with the good bacteria? Or is it growing out of control? This is extremely difficult to assess. Even lab test results are often unclear about it, even in very severe states of overgrowth.

Most medical doctors do not recognize candida as a problem in normal people. However, they recognize thrush in an AIDS victim and treat it immediately. But since most people's immune systems never become so compromised, the kind of extreme overgrowth of yeast seen in an AIDS patient is rarely seen in the normal population.

> He had heard that Hezekiah had been very sick and that he had recovered.
>
> —ISAIAH 39:1, NLT

Nevertheless, even when candida overgrowth is not life-threatening, still it is able to produce the symptoms recognized as candidiasis or the yeast syndrome.

Most nutritional doctors will diagnose candidiasis based on a detailed medical history and a yeast questionnaire. Occasionally he or she will request that a comprehensive digestive stool analysis be taken. This careful examination of the stool helps your doctor to evaluate how well your food is being digested and absorbed, to check for parasites, to identify the presence of beneficial and pathogenic bacteria and to identify excessive yeast overgrowth.

I routinely have my patients complete the yeast questionnaire developed by Dr. William Crook.[2]

A **BIBLE CURE** Health Tip

What About You?

Would you like to know if your own health problems are yeast-related? Then answer the questions below and add up your points to see how you stack up.[3]

1. Have you taken tetracycline or other antibiotics for acne for one month or longer?....................................25

2. Have you ever taken other broad-spectrum antibiotics for respiratory, urinary or other infections for two months or longer, or in short courses four or more times in one year?................ 20

3. Have you ever taken a broad-spectrum antibiotic (even a single course)?..6

4. Have you ever been bothered by persistent prostatitis, vaginitis or other problems affecting your reproductive organs?........25

5. Have you been pregnant...
   One time?.. 3
   Two or more times?............................... 5

6. Have you taken birth control pills...
   For six months to two years?........................ 8
   For more than two years?........................... 15

7. Have you taken prednisone or other cortisone-type drugs...
   For two weeks or less?............................. 6
   For more than two weeks?.......................... 15

8. Does exposure to perfumes, insecticides, fabric shop odors and other chemicals provoke...
   Mild symptoms?.................................... 5
   Moderate to severe symptoms?....................... 20

9. Are your symptoms worse on damp, muggy days or
   in moldy places? 20

10. Have you had athlete's foot, ringworm, "jock-itch" or other
    chronic infections of the skin or nails?
    Mild to moderate? 10
    Severe or persistent? 20

11. Do you crave sugar? 10

12. Do you crave breads?....................................10

13. Do you crave alcoholic beverages?.........................10

14. Does tobacco smoke really bother you? 10

If you are a woman and scored over 180, or a man and scored over 140, yeast-connected problems are almost certainly present.

If you are a woman and scored 120–180, or a man and scored 90–140, yeast-connected health problems are probably present.

If you are a woman and scored 60–119, or a man and scored 40–89, yeast-connected health problems are possibly present.

If you are a woman and scored less than 60, or a man and scored less than 40, yeast-connected health problems are less likely present.

KNOWING THE SCORE

So, how did you score? Knowing where you stand is essential in your battle against yeast syndrome. Whether you scored higher or lower than you expected really doesn't matter. By reading this book, you hold in your hands valuable keys to overcoming the distressing yeast syndrome forever. Let's take a look at your body's main defense team against candida: your incredible immune system.

YOUR INCREDIBLE DEFENSE TEAM

It's vital for you to improve immune function to overcome the yeast syndrome. The immune system is how your body protects itself against yeast, fungi, bacteria, viruses, cancer cells and other foreign invaders. Chances are that if you have chronic candida, then you may also have a depressed immune system.

If the cells of your immune system formed a football team, the white blood cells would play defense. White blood cells are actually produced in the bone marrow, but they are found in large numbers in the blood and in lymphoid tissues. The lymphoid tissues include the thymus, spleen and lymph nodes.

The thymus gland is the quarterback—it's a main player in the immune system's defense against yeast. That's why strengthening your thymus can help you win against candida.

The thymus is a small gland located under the upper breastbone, which produces helper T-cells that rally other white blood cells into action. When a helper T-cell recognizes that an invader like yeast is attacking the body, it signals to B-cells to make antibodies that are specific for that particular foreign invader. Antibodies then destroy the invader.

> LORD, your discipline is good, for it leads to life and health.
> —ISAIAH 38:16, NLT

Other T-cells that are produced by the thymus include suppressor T-cells, which help to keep the B-cells in check. This prevents them from overproducing antibodies. Natural killer cells are also stimulated by helper T-cells to kill tumor cells.

You can see how important the thymus gland is. When the thymus is weak, not only can yeast overgrow, but your body also becomes more susceptible to viral and bacterial infections. You also become more susceptible to cancer. The thymus is also important in protecting your body from autoimmune diseases like rheumatoid arthritis and lupus.

Building up your immune system is a powerful and natural way to help your body score a winning touchdown against the yeast syndrome. In the following chapters we'll address some powerful ways to fortify your immune system's strength and help to free you from candida forever!

CONCLUSION

Yeast syndrome is not a chronic battle that you cannot win. It's not a life sentence of pain, distress and embarrassment. God is granting a treasure of wisdom and good sense to you about the yeast syndrome so that you can understand how it works and how you can work with your body to defeat it.

Wisdom, however, is just the first key. In the following chapters we will explore powerful ways you can strike back at the root of candida and destroy its hold on your body forever. By following the spiritual and natural keys presented within the following pages, you can restore your body's natural balance and reclaim your health.

A **BIBLE CURE** Prayer for You

Dear God, I thank You for the wisdom You are providing for me as the first key to becoming free of the yeast syndrome forever. I acknowledge that nothing is greater than You—You are higher and greater than all that concerns me physically, mentally and spiritually. I believe that You truly and genuinely care about all of my health concerns, and I thank You for Your great compassion. In Jesus' name, amen.

A **BIBLE CURE** *Prescription*

Did you take the yeast syndrome test in this chapter? If so, what was your score?

_____

What symptoms of yeast do you have on a chronic basis?

_____

_____

_____

_____

_____

_____

_____

Do you believe that God genuinely cares about everything about you—including all of your health issues?

_____

_____

_____

_____

_____

_____

_____

_____

_____

_____

Chapter 24

RESTORE YOUR
HEALTH WITH NUTRITION

YOU HAVE ALREADY seen that the yeast syndrome can sweep through your body like a plague, robbing your energy and ravaging your health. But God is a restorer, and He promises to restore you back to health and vigor. The Bible says, "For I will restore you to health" (Jer. 30:17, NASB).

God does indeed promise full restoration. Again, the Bible says, "Then I will make up to you for the years that the swarming locust has eaten, the creeping locust, the stripping locust, and the gnawing locust" (Joel 2:25, NASB).

Let's look at a powerful Bible cure key to your total restoration and recovery: nutrition.

DIETARY FACTORS YOU SHOULD KNOW

In order to experience recovery from yeast overgrowth, it's critically important to make some changes to your diet. Certain dietary factors promote candida overgrowth that you can control.

You will need to adhere strictly to a special diet for a period of time in order to experience full restoration of your body's natural balance. How long will depend upon the severity of your yeast syndrome, as candida ranges from extremely mild to very severe.

> He fills my life with good things. My youth is renewed like the eagle's!
> —PSALM 103:5, NLT

The majority of patients suffering from candida will need to stay on the diet for three months. Patients with severe candidiasis will need to stay on the diet six months to one year, and patients with mild candida may need to stay on the diet only one to two months.

Let's take a look at some dietary factors that promote yeast overgrowth.

YOUR SWEET TOOTH

If you have a sweet tooth, you may have to wait to satisfy it. Believe it or not, the average American takes in about 150 pounds of sugar per person per year! Sugar-rich foods are the single most important contributing factor to candida overgrowth. That's why sugar must be strictly avoided for a season of time so that your body has a chance to reclaim its natural balance.

What you eat will determine how well your immune system is able to function. A high-sugar diet will impair immunity. This means all sugars, including the following:

- White sugar
- Brown sugar
- Syrups
- Honey
- Fructose

- Glucose
- Maltose
- Maple sugar
- Molasses
- Date sugar

Even the sugars found in fruit juices and high-sugar vegetable juices like carrot juice must be omitted. Fruits should be omitted for the first three weeks of the yeast-free diet. The herbal sweetener Stevia is an excellent alternative to sugar. Also, the new sugar substitute Splenda is acceptable in moderation.

MILK PRODUCTS AND YOU

Milk and milk products contain lactose, which also encourages candida growth. Small amounts of butter are acceptable for most individuals with less-severe cases of candida.

Lactose-free yogurt and kefir are exceptions. They are actually good for you, for they contain good bacteria that help to restore bacteria in the bowel. Some people always make it a point to eat yogurt when taking antibiotics and certain other drugs that we will discuss later on. This can be especially helpful before yeast grows out of control. However, avoid kefir and yogurt that contain sugar, fruit or lactose, since these products will feed the yeast.

So, What About Fruit?

Fruit should be avoided for the first three weeks. After that you may reintroduce the less sweet fruits. Eat fruit by itself thirty minutes before your meals. Here's a list of fruit you can reintroduce into your diet:

- Lemons
- Limes
- Apples
- Kiwi
- Blackberries

- Grapefruits
- Watermelon
- Raspberries
- Strawberries
- Blueberries

Here are some sweet fruits to avoid:

- Dried fruits
- Bananas
- Cherries
- Grapes
- Peaches
- Plums

- Oranges
- Cantaloupe
- Honeydew
- Mangoes
- Pineapple

Dealing With Carbs

Most of us love carbs, especially when it comes to breads and snack foods. Nevertheless, while you are working with your body to restore it to natural balance, closely watching what carbohydrates you eat is vitally important.

Candida loves refined carbohydrates and thrives on them, so they actually become food for the candida rather than for you. By decreasing these refined carbohydrates, you will slow down the rate of multiplication of yeast cells. Here's a list of refined carbs to avoid:

- White bread
- Pasta
- Muffins
- Pancakes

- Most breakfast cereals
- Potato chips
- Corn chips
- White crackers

In addition to these food items, you will need to decrease your consumption of both packaged and processed foods. Most of these foods are highly processed. Refined sugar is added to this list as well. These foods are a perfect source to help yeast to multiply. Sugar and highly processed foods depress the immune system. All of these foods also have a high glycemic index. The glycemic index of a food is simply how rapidly a food causes the blood sugar to rise.[1]

CARBS YOU CAN CHOOSE

Some less-refined carbohydrates are actually good for you and highly desirable. As long as the following foods have not been refined, they are safe for you.

- Oats
- Millet bread
- Brown rice
- Spelt pasta

- Buckwheat
- Quinoa
- Amaranth
- Spelt

WHAT ABOUT WHOLE WHEAT?

If you have mild candida overgrowth, whole wheat may be fine for your diet. However, if your candida score fell into the moderate to severe range, then wheat is probably off limits for you, and you may be unable to tolerate whole wheat. If after eating whole-wheat products you develop bloating, belching, gas, drowsiness, irritability, mood changes or other symptoms of candida, you should avoid all wheat products for at least three months. Also, most whole-wheat products such as bread are made with yeast and therefore should be avoided.

Wheat is high in the protein gluten, and many individuals with candida overgrowth are gluten-sensitive. For such individuals, eating whole-wheat products may worsen their candida.

Therefore, if symptoms of candida occur after eating wheat products, stop eating grains for three months, and then reintroduce them slowly back into your diet, combining them primarily with vegetables.

Oats also contain gluten, but in lower amounts than wheat. Oats may need to be avoided if symptoms occur.

OTHER FOODS TO AVOID

Foods with yeast and mold

Avoid foods with high amounts of yeast or mold in them. These include all cheeses and most breads, pastries and other baked goods containing yeast. Yeast- or mold-containing foods do not make candida grow; however, they cause symptoms such as bloating, gas, belching, irritability and other symptoms because many are allergic or sensitive to yeast products.

Some condiments

Avoid condiments and sauces that contain yeast such as mustard, ketchup, barbecue sauce, soy sauce, steak sauce and Worcestershire sauce. Other condiments high in yeast include pickles, sauerkraut, horseradish, relishes, miso, tempeh and tamari.

If you have mild symptoms of candida, these foods should be avoided for one to two months. Most patients should avoid them for three months. If you have severe symptoms of candida, you should avoid them six months to a year.

Vinegary foods

Foods containing vinegar should also be avoided. These include nearly all salad dressings, mayonnaise and mayonnaise products. Raw, unfiltered apple cider vinegar is one exception, however. If a patient with yeast has no symptoms of candida (such as bloating, belching, gas, irritability or mood changes), he may tolerate this very well because apple cider vinegar actually contains good bacteria that fight yeast proliferation. However, some patients with candida overgrowth cannot take any forms of vinegar.

Preserved and processed meats

Some specially prepared and preserved meats can be high in yeast. They include pickled and smoked meats and fish, sausages, corned beef, hot dogs, bacon, ham and pastrami.

Nuts

Nuts are often high in mold, especially when they are not stored in airtight containers in the refrigerator or freezer. To prevent nuts and seeds from getting moldy, purchase them in their shells and crack and eat them as you desire. However, avoid peanuts and cashews since they usually have a higher mold content. Patients with candida are usually allergic or sensitive to mold.

Mushrooms

Mold, as well as yeast foods, causes symptoms when a person is allergic or sensitive to yeast products. Avoid all types of mushrooms since these are fungi, and yeast is simply a form of fungus.

Leftovers

Discard all leftovers after a day or two since they tend to grow mold.

Alcoholic beverages

Alcoholic beverages (such as beer) contain a high content of yeast and should be avoided.

Allergy-causing foods

Finally, the last group of foods that you must avoid is allergy-causing foods. Commonly, food allergies involve the following foods:

- Eggs
- Dairy products
- Wheat
- Corn
- Yeast
- Chocolate
- Citrus fruits

To determine if you have food allergies or sensitivities, you can have a RAST test. For more information on food allergies, read my book *The Bible Cure for Allergies.*

WHAT CAN I EAT?

Now that we have talked about all the foods that you should avoid, let's talk about all the foods that you can eat. Vegetables are one of the most important foods for a person with candida overgrowth. You should eat a minimum of three to five servings of vegetables a day.

VIRTUOUS VEGETABLES

Even though it's best to eat vegetables raw, you can lightly steam or stir-fry them as well. You can also make many varieties of delicious vegetable soup.

If you have candida, just avoid these veggies: potatoes, mushrooms and sweet potatoes. Potatoes and sweet potatoes have a high glycemic index, which feeds yeast. Mushrooms are a yeast food.

Eat at least three to five servings of the following vegetables a day (a serving equals either 1 cup cooked or 2 cups raw):

- Artichokes
- Avocados
- Green beans
- Broccoli
- Cabbage
- Cauliflower
- Chard
- Cucumbers
- Garlic
- Lettuce (all types)
- Onions
- Parsnips
- Green bell peppers
- Radishes
- Soybeans
- Sprouts
- Squash (yellow, summer)
- Water chestnuts

- Asparagus
- Beans
- Beet greens
- Brussels sprouts
- Carrots
- Celery
- Eggplant
- Greens (kale, chard, mustard, collard, spinach, turnip)
- Parsley
- Peppers
- Hot chili peppers
- Snow peas
- Spinach
- Alfalfa sprouts
- Tomatoes
- Turnips
- Zucchini

(You can make a delicious soup with a combination of these vegetables.)

Beans or legumes are high in protein and have about the same amount

of calories as grains. They are also very high in f
beans, black-eyed peas, garbanzo beans, kidn
beans, pinto beans, red beans, soybeans and sp
are combined with grains, they form a comple

POWERFUL PROTEINS

Meats, poultry and fish do not feed candida. However, some animals
are fed antibiotics, which remain in meat and can cause yeast to proliferate. That's why it is important for you to choose meat and poultry
that are free of antibiotics, such as free-range beef and chicken.

Try to eat fish at least three times a week. Choose fatty fish such as
salmon, herring, mackerel, halibut or sardines since they have a high
content of omega-3 fatty acids. You may also have lamb or veal.

EGGSXACTLY!

Finally, you may eat two to three servings of eggs each week, unless
you are allergic to them. Just be sure to cook them well.

FABULOUS FATS

The right fats add zest to your meals, and they are very healthy for
your body. The fabulous fats allowed on the diet include extra-virgin
olive oil, flaxseed oil, organic butter and cold-pressed vegetable oil
such as safflower oil.

A **BIBLE CURE** *Recipe*

Really Good Salad Dressing

Some of my patients have complained that they cannot eat salads on this
diet because it contains vinegar. Well, here's a salad dressing you can make
that is really good!

> 2 Tbsp. extra-virgin olive oil
> 1 Tbsp. purified water
> 1 Tbsp. freshly squeezed lemon juice (or apple cider vinegar if you have
>   no symptoms with it)
> 1 tsp. tarragon

garlic salt

ρ. parsley flakes

⌐ash of pepper

Dash of salt

2–3 drops Stevia (sweeten to taste)

Shake in cruet or jar. Pour over salad.

MEAL PLANNING FOR THE CANDIDA DIET

Here are some helpful meal suggestions to get you started on your candida diet.

Breakfast

Day 1

- Egg omelet with sliced onion, tomatoes and peppers
- 1 slice millet, spelt or yeast-free rye toast or rice toast
- 1 pat organic butter

Day 2

- Old-fashioned oatmeal with cinnamon and almonds (cooked in water instead of milk)
- Sweeten with Stevia or Splenda
- 1 pat organic butter

Day 3

- Toasted rice or millet bread
- Top with almond butter spread

Day 4

- 2 scrambled eggs
- Toasted millet bread
- Brown rice
- 1 pat organic butter

Day 5

- Sunflower and sesame seeds mixed with hot oat bran cereal

Day 6

- Oat, rice, spelt or amaranth pancakes

- Raspberries, blackberries, strawberries or blueberries

- Sprinkle with Stevia or Splenda (This one must be eaten three weeks after the beginning of the candida program since fruits are introduced at this time.)

Day 7

- Organic plain low-fat yogurt or kefir with 1 tsp. acidophilus powder

- Fresh berries

- Sweeten with Stevia or Splenda (Again, this should be added three weeks after the beginning of the program. Also, realize that some people may not tolerate fruit with pancakes, so they may need to eat it thirty minutes before eating the pancakes or the yogurt.)

Lunches or Dinners

Day 1

- Baked, broiled or grilled chicken

- Brown rice

- Lima beans

Day 2

- Broiled, baked or grilled fish

- Green beans

- Broccoli

Day 3

- Turkey

- Lima beans

- Asparagus

- 1 slice millet bread

- 1 pat organic butter

Day 4

- 4 oz. free-range, lean filet mignon

- Brown rice

- Asparagus

Day 5

- Tuna fish sandwich

- Millet bread

- Lettuce, tomato and onions

Day 6

- Cornish hen

- Black-eyed peas

- Cooked carrots

Day 7

- Grilled salmon

- Green peas

- Broccoli

Feel free to add a salad to any one of these dinners. In addition, add all the vegetables you want. Just avoid croutons, cheese and most dressings. You may use the salad dressing recipe on page 239. Also, you may eat vegetable soup with any vegetables that are listed.

So, How Long?

If you have candida, expect to go on this program for one to six months, depending upon the severity of your symptoms. If your symptoms are severe, maintain the program for six months. If moderate, go on the program for three months. If your symptoms are mild, one to two months will be all the time you need. Go off the program when you have been symptom free at least one to three months.

Eating to Improve Your Immune System

Even after you've completed the candida diet regimen and your yeast is under control, you will still want to continue to strengthen your immune system through ongoing good nutrition. A strong immune system will overcome yeast attacks and protect your body from future invasions.

A diet high in saturated fat, such as animal fats, butter, cheese and whole milk, impairs immune function. But whole natural foods such as vegetables, fruits, whole grains, beans, seeds and nuts will help to improve the immune system. Also, omega-3 fatty acids, such as what is found in fatty fish such as salmon and mackerel, strengthens the immune system. Flaxseed oil, evening primrose oil and black currant oil all help to improve the immune system as well.

Eating enough protein helps your immune system by increasing the production of antibodies that fight off bacteria and other invaders. And be sure to drink plenty of clean, filtered water—at least two quarts every day. But avoid chlorinated tap water that destroys friendly bacteria and can cause an overgrowth of yeast.

A Word About Food Allergies

If you scored high on the test for yeast syndrome, I encourage you to get tested for food allergies and sensitivities since they can play an integral role in the development of yeast syndrome.

Many individuals have food allergies and food sensitivities. You could be one of them. It's critically important to identify, eliminate or desensitize food allergies to properly restore immune function. Food allergies cause food that should be nourishing our bodies to create allergic reactions in our GI tracts.

WHAT'S LEAKY GUT?

Food allergies are often related to a problem called "leaky gut." Leaky gut occurs when the lining of our intestines, which is supposed to absorb food and act as a barrier to keep out invading organisms, lies down on the job. This can happen when candida damages our GI tract.

> But those who trust in the LORD will find new strength. They will soar high on wings like eagles. They will run and not grow weary. They will walk and not faint.
>
> —ISAIAH 40:31, NLT

Leaky gut opens a door for bacteria, yeast, viruses, parasites and undigested food molecules, as well as yeast and their toxic waste products, to enter the bloodstream. They then begin circulating. The partially digested food molecules activate the immune system, creating food allergies and food sensitivities. This further damages the lining of the GI tract, creating symptoms of fatigue, rashes, diarrhea, abdominal pain, memory loss, arthritis, autoimmune diseases, psoriasis and acne.

When yeast overgrowth damages the intestinal walls, it becomes difficult for friendly bacteria to recolonize the area. Pretty soon large molecules of incompletely digested food protein and yeast by-products begin to enter into the bloodstream, provoking immune responses. This in turn creates food allergies or sensitivities to numerous commonly eaten foods. It also causes food allergies or sensitivities to practically all yeast products such as mushrooms, soy sauce and breads with yeast.

You can see that a leaky gut creates a vicious cycle. When you eat a food that you're allergic or sensitive to, or when you eat a yeast-type food, the GI tract becomes inflamed and damages—and even destroys—cells in the intestines due to allergic reactions occurring in the lining of the intestines. As this process continues, it damages the intestinal tract even further and creates symptoms of bloating, gas, discomfort, diarrhea, spastic colon and nausea.

To rid your intestinal tract of yeast you must strengthen your immune system, repair the damaged intestinal tract, avoid foods that feed yeast or that you are allergic to, kill the yeast overgrowth with herbs and medication that we will look at later, repopulate the GI tract with good bacteria and at the same time sweep the excessive yeast overgrowth out with high-fiber foods.

Clearing up food allergies is extremely important in overcoming candida. I discuss this in detail in *The Bible Cure for Allergies*.

FIBER FACTS

When you have a buildup of yeast and bacteria in your body, detoxifying is essential to restore you back to health.

One of the most important means of detoxifying the body is to have regular bowel movements on a daily basis, which means you must eat plenty of fiber and drink plenty of water.

You need at least 25–35 grams of fiber every day. The fiber intake of most Americans is far below this number. When you are dealing with an overgrowth of yeast, fiber helps to eliminate yeast so that it is not reabsorbed back into the body.

During the first week of your candida program, candida die-off reactions usually occur. When a yeast cell dies, it becomes food for another yeast cell, which tends to encourage the yeast colonies that are still present. The internal fluids of the dead yeast cells are feeding these yeast colonies. Therefore, it is critically important to eliminate these dead yeast cells through adequate fiber intake.

WHAT YOU NEED TO KNOW ABOUT FIBER

Two types of fiber are available to you: soluble and insoluble fiber.

Soluble fiber

Examples of soluble fiber are listed as follows:

- Psyllium seed
- Fruit pectin
- Oat bran
- Rice bran

Soluble fiber actually feeds the good bacteria that live in the intestines. It ferments to produce short-chain fatty acids. These fatty acids nourish the cells in the large intestines, thus stimulating healing.

You need to get adequate amounts of soluble fiber, but not too much. Too much soluble fiber causes an overgrowth of intestinal bacteria, which in turn can create more problems for you by increasing bacterial toxins.

Insoluble fiber

Insoluble fiber is found in wheat bran and methylcellulose, which is a tasteless powder that gets swollen and gummy when wet. However, I don't recommend wheat bran for individuals with yeast overgrowth since many are sensitive to wheat products. Methylcellulose inactivates many toxins in the GI tract. It also stops bad bacteria and parasites from attacking the intestines, and it protects a person from developing increased gut permeability, which is worsening of the leaky gut.

To win your battle against candida you will need to eat high-fiber foods and take fiber supplements. A good fiber supplement is Ultrafiber by Metagenics, which contains barley bran, rice bran, cellulose, apple fiber, beet fiber and apple pectin. Take two scoops at bedtime with 8 ounces of water. You may also take two scoops upon awakening with a chlorophyll drink, which will be discussed later.

IMPROVING DIGESTION

Not only are the foods you eat important in your battle against candida, but the way you eat your foods is just as important. Let's take a look at some ways you can assist your body by improving digestion.

- Drink a beverage about thirty minutes before eating.

- Digestion actually starts in the mouth, so it's critically important to mix the food you're eating with saliva. Your saliva contains enzymes that help to digest starches.

- Chew food slowly and thoroughly to break down the food properly. When it finally reaches the small intestines, it will be further broken down and assimilated more easily into the body.

- Take special care to chew meats and other protein foods extra thoroughly so that they can be digested properly in the stomach.

- Take one or two digestive enzymes with each meal.
  You may also take a hydrochloric acid supplement,
  one to two with each meal as recommended by your
  nutritionist. These may be purchased at a health food
  store. If you have a history of ulcer disease, gastritis
  or burning abdominal pains, consult your nutritional
  doctor prior to taking either of these supplements.

Believe it or not, if you have candida overgrowth and poor digestion, your body may be using most of your energy to digest your food.
That's why you often feel exhausted.

WHAT TO EAT WITH WHAT

Food combining has a powerful effect on digestion also. Food combining is especially important for candida sufferers. Here are some
important food combining tips:

- Meats and proteins should not be eaten together with
  high-starch foods.

- Meats and proteins can be eaten with low-starch vegetables such as green beans, broccoli, cauliflower, asparagus and salads.

- Low-starch vegetables can also be eaten together with
  starchy vegetables such as potatoes and whole grains.

- Fruits should be eaten approximately thirty minutes
  before a meal and should be eaten alone.

CONCLUSION

Even if yeast has swept through your system like a plague of hungry
locusts, stripping your intestines, gnawing away at your intestinal
walls and breaking down your health by creeping into every organ
system in your body, you are being armed with important and valuable weapons to defeat it. By giving you these vital keys, God has
already begun to bring you full restoration. Believe God when He
promises to restore to you the years that the plague of locusts has
eaten. (See Joel 2:25.) God's promises are sure. He will not fail you!

A **BIBLE CURE** *Prayer for You*

Dear God, thank You for beginning the process of total restoration for my body. Even though the yeast syndrome has attacked my body, Your power and wisdom are greater than every attack and every disease. Give me special divinely ordained grace to undergo a time of special dieting for candida. And help me to develop lifestyle changes that will set me free from the yeast syndrome attacks for the rest of my days. In Jesus' name, amen.

A **BIBLE CURE** Prescription

This diet is for the initial phase of your program and will be the strictest during this time. Candida feeds on certain foods, and these foods will need to be eliminated for a season.

Check the foods you will stop eating until your body's balance is restored.

❏ No sugar of any kind—white sugar, brown sugar, honey, molasses, barley, malt, rice syrup, etc.

❏ No artificial sweeteners—Sweet 'N Low, NutraSweet, Equal, etc. (Stevia is allowed.)

❏ No fruit juice of any kind for the first three months, then gradually added back into diet if tolerated.

❏ No fruit of any kind for the first three weeks, then gradually added back into diet starting with low-glycemic fruits such as apples, kiwi, berries, grapefruit, lemons and limes.

❏ No dairy food of any kind—milk, cheese, cottage cheese, ice cream, sour cream, etc. (A small amount of organic butter, and yogurt and kefir with no lactose, sugar or fruit are acceptable.)

❏ No gluten grains of any kind found in wheat, rye, white or pumpernickel breads, or found in pastry, crackers, etc. (Rice bread found in the frozen section of the health food store is a good replacement. Millet bread is also acceptable.) Oats contain less gluten, however, and may not be tolerated by those with severe candida.

❏ No foods containing yeast

❏ No breads or other bakery products containing yeast

❏ No alcoholic beverages of any kind

❏ No commercially prepared foods containing yeast

❏ No dry roasted nuts (Nuts in the shell—other than peanuts or cashews—are acceptable. The shell protects them from molding.)

❏ No vinegar and vinegar-containing foods with the possible exception of raw, unfiltered apple cider vinegar in those with mild candida.

❏ No soy sauce, tamari or natural root beer.

❏ No vitamin and mineral supplements containing yeast

❏ No pickled foods or smoked, dried or cured meats, including bacon

❏ No deep-fried foods of any kind

❏ No mushrooms

Chapter 25

RENEW YOUR
BODY WITH SUPPLEMENTS

E VEN IF YOUR body feels completely depleted by candida attack, God promises to renew your health and strength. The Bible says, "Bless the LORD, O my soul, and forget not all His benefits: Who forgives all your iniquities, who heals all your diseases, who redeems your life from destruction, who crowns you with lovingkindness and tender mercies, who satisfies your mouth with good things, so that your youth is renewed like the eagle's" (Ps. 103:2–5, NKJV).

Renewal comes from God. The Word of God declares, "But those who wait on the LORD shall renew their strength; they shall mount up with wings as eagles, they shall run and not be weary, and they shall walk and not faint" (Isa. 40:31, NKJV).

Renewal comes from God, but often He uses natural methods to bring health and healing to you. He has filled the earth with many natural substances that, used with God's wisdom, can become instruments of His healing touch. For whether healing comes supernaturally or naturally, all healing comes from God, and all restoration is the benefit of His blessing.

Let's take a look at some of the powerful, natural herbs and other supplements for the third dynamic key of this Bible cure.

SUPPLEMENTS,
HERBS AND MEDICATIONS

A number of natural herbs and supplements are powerfully effective against candida. In addition to your special candida diet, begin supplementing with sources of good bacteria. The lining of your GI tract has been a war zone and will need special healing, and any parasitic infestations you may have must also be addressed.

Let's look at some supplements that can help.

Garlic

One of the most important supplements for controlling yeast overgrowth is garlic. Allicin, the active ingredient in garlic, has powerful anti-fungal activity.

Take 500 milligrams of garlic three times a day.

Goldenseal

Goldenseal is included in the same family with Oregon grape and barberry. They are all in the berberines family. These potent natural substances contain extremely effective antifungal agents. These special agents actually activate macrophages, which are a type of white blood cell.

Berberines help to clear out bacterial overgrowth in the small intestines, which commonly accompanies yeast overgrowth. Berberines also halt the bacterial and yeast enzymes that aggravate leaky gut. Many patients with chronic candidiasis have diarrhea. Berberines are also able to control diarrhea in many cases.

Take 500 milligrams of goldenseal three times a day for at least a month.

Grapefruit seed extract

Grapefruit seed extract, otherwise known as citrus extract, is a great supplement. It effectively kills both the candida and the parasite giardia, which may be associated with candida in some cases. However, it usually takes several months to eliminate the parasites.

Take 100–200 milligrams of grapefruit seed extract three times a day.

Caprylic acid

Caprylic acid is a long-chain fatty acid found in coconuts. It's extremely toxic to yeast, yet safe for humans. To be effective it must be taken in a time-released capsule.

Take 1000 milligrams of a time-released preparation with each meal.

Oil of oregano

Oil of oregano is a very good antifungal agent. It's more than one hundred times more potent than caprylic acid. I recommend oregano oil tablets from the nutritional company Biotics.

Take three 50-milligram tablets of oregano three times a day.

Tanalbit

Tanalbit is a plant extract that destroys yeast, including the spores, without harming good bacteria. It also contains natural tannins, which have intestinal antiseptic properties.

Take three capsules three times a day with each meal.

Chlorophyll supplements (green food)

Chlorophyll supplements, otherwise known as green food supplements, detoxify the colon and pack a powerful punch against candida. They boost the immune system as well. Chlorophyll keeps yeast and bacteria from spreading, and it even encourages the growth of friendly bacteria.

High-chlorophyll foods include wheat grass, barley grass, alfalfa, chlorella, spiralina and blue/green algae. All of these are obtained in Divine Health Green Superfood. (This is a supplement that I produce. It can be purchased by contacting my office or through the Internet at www.drcolbert.com.) These high-chlorophyll foods are very nutrient-dense and are excellent sources of essential amino acids, vitamins, minerals, essential fatty acids and phytonutrients.

I recommend one scoop one to two times a day mixed with the fiber supplement. I find it best to take this upon awakening. Do not take Green Superfood in the evening since it is very stimulating and may cause insomnia. However, all the ingredients are natural and contain no stimulants such as caffeine or ephedra.

I personally start my morning as soon as I awaken with two scoops of Ultrafiber, one scoop of Green Superfood, one-half fresh, squeezed lemon or lime and 8 ounces of water. I place this in a shaker cup, shake it for about twenty seconds and then drink. Stevia can be added to sweeten it.

High-chloropyll foods not only boost the immune system, but they also help to improve both digestion and elimination.

CANDIDA MEDICATIONS

In addition to supplements and herbs, I commonly use medications to control candida.

Nystatin

Nystatin is an antifungal antibiotic that is able to kill a wide variety of different types of yeast. Most folks can take it without side effects. Nystatin tends to stay in the GI tract and do its work instead of being absorbed into other parts of the body. Nystatin is even safe for infants to use. But because Nystatin is poorly absorbed, it may not be as effective for candida that has attacked the entire body.

Ask your doctor about prescribing this medication for you.

A CANDIDA-BUSTING COCKTAIL

For a very mild case of candida, I simply recommend 1000 milligrams of caprylic acid three times a day with meals and 500 milligrams of garlic three times a day.

Here's what I prescribe to those experiencing a mild to moderate case of candida:

- Nystatin, 1,000,000 units three times a day
- Caprylic acid, 1000 mg. three times a day
- Garlic, 500 mg. three times a day

If the yeast problem does not go away, I may add any of the following:

- Grapefruit seed extract, 200 mg. three times a day
- Oil of oregano, three 50-mg. tablets three times a day
- Tanalbit, three capsules three times a day
- Goldenseal, 500 mg. three times a day

If the infection is very severe I will often use the medication Diflucan.

Diflucan

Diflucan is so powerful that a single 150-milligram tablet can treat a vaginal candida infection. If your candida overgrowth is severe, you may need to take Diflucan anywhere from a few weeks up to as long as a month.

There are many other medications for yeast available. However, I believe that these are the safest ones presently available.

DETOXING FOR DYNAMIC RESULTS

When candida herbs or medications are taken, yeast die-off reactions commonly occur. This die-off reaction is called a "Herxheimer Reaction." When your body begins rapidly killing off the candida, it may absorb large amounts of the yeast cell particles and toxins.

If you are experiencing this reaction, these symptoms may occur: gas, headaches, fatigue, muscle aches, joint aches, sinus congestion, sore throat, rashes, dizziness and even depression. These symptoms seldom last longer than a few days or up to a week after starting yeast herbs or medications.

> Restore us, O LORD, and bring us back to you again! Give us back the joys we once had!
>
> —LAMENTATIONS 5:21, NLT

The answer to this sloughing off of dead yeast is detoxing. As your body goes through this process, detoxing will help your body cleanse itself from this increase of toxins.

LIVER DETOXIFICATION

Not only does candida overgrowth affect the immune system and GI tract, but it also has a very profound impact upon the liver as well.

Liver detoxification is occurring continually in the body. However, many times the body's detoxification pathways are overwhelmed by yeast, toxins produced by yeast, leaky gut, food allergies and so on. Therefore, herbs and supplements are critically important for supporting and improving liver detoxification.

Liver detoxification takes place in two phases.

Phase 1

During Phase 1 detoxification, destructive toxins are burned or oxidized, which causes them to become more soluble in water. Let me explain. The liver is like a large filter and is designed to remove toxic material such as drugs, chemicals, dead cells, toxins, yeast bacteria and other microorganisms. The liver has two main detoxification pathways for breaking down and removing these toxic substances. The pathways are called Phase 1 and Phase 2 detoxification. Phase 1 converts a toxin to a less harmful toxin. This is done through chemical reactions, which can in turn produce large amounts of free radicals that can further damage the liver cells.

This process tends to produce free radicals. Free radicals can also damage liver cells, and they can damage the lining of the intestines as the free radicals are excreted through the bile and then dumped into the GI tract. This in turn can aggravate leaky gut.

Antioxidants never work alone. They work together to help to recycle one another. So I recommend taking a comprehensive antioxidant formula that contains plenty of vitamin E, vitamin C, lipoic acid, coenzyme Q_{10}, grape seed and pine bark extract, beta carotene and the minerals copper, zinc, manganese, selenium and sulfur. These can be obtained in Divine Health Multivitamins and Divine Health Antioxidants.

> Do not rejoice over me, O my enemy. Though I fall I will rise; though I dwell in darkness, the LORD is a light for me.
> —MICAH 7:8, NASB

Phase 2

The other phase of liver detoxification is Phase 2 detoxification. In this phase, the chemicals that are oxidized during Phase 1 are joined to an amino acid or another compound to render it less harmful. As the toxin is joined to the amino acid, it becomes water soluble so that it can be excreted from the body by the bile or in the urine.

The most important amino acids for Phase 2 detoxification are cysteine, taurine and methionine, which are sulfur-containing amino acids. Eggs, garlic, onions, cruciferous veggies (cabbage, broccoli, cauliflower, Brussels sprouts), fish, poultry and meats are good sources of sulfur, which aids in Phase 2 detoxification. Choose free-range meat and chicken. At lease one sulfur-containing food should be eaten daily. Cysteine and methionine are also converted into glutathione, which is a potent detoxifier of the liver. It is also an antioxidant.

To assist your body in Phase 2 detoxification, I recommend the following:

- Take N-acetyl cysteine, otherwise known as NAC, and taurine. These supplements will help replenish glutathione stores, which protect the liver from damage from drugs and other toxins. I recommend 500 milligrams of NAC and 500 milligrams of taurine daily.

- Eat at least one serving a week of cruciferous vegetables such as broccoli, cauliflower, Brussels sprouts and cabbage to help to improve liver detoxification.

Restoring Life to Your Liver

Several other supplements will restore your liver to health and vitality.

Milk thistle

Milk thistle contains a bioflavonoid called silymarin that also protects the liver against toxins. Silymarin—the active ingredient in milk thistle—prevents the depletion of glutathione. I recommend 100–200 milligrams of silymarin three times a day.

Glutathione

Glutathione is the most important antioxidant that enables the liver to detoxify. Silymarin can increase the level of glutathione in the liver up to 35 percent. The combination of milk thistle (silymarin) and N-acetyl cysteine (NAC) is extremely important in restoring glutathione levels and thus in protecting and restoring normal liver function. As above, I recommend 100–200 milligrams of silymarin (milk thistle) three times a day and 500 milligrams of NAC once a day.

Lipoic acid

Lipoic acid is also important in increasing the levels of glutathione. I recommend 100–200 milligrams of lipoic acid three times a day for severe candidiasis, and 50–100 milligrams three times a day for moderate candida.

If you have mild candida, all you usually need is a multivitamin and antioxidant formula. If you have severe candidiasis, you will need the multivitamin and antioxidants in addition to supplements of milk thistle, NAC, taurine and extra lipoic acid.

RESTORING FRIENDLY BACTERIA

When we think of bacteria, most of us think of something negative, such as a bacterial infection. But as we saw earlier, bacteria are not all bad. As a matter of fact, much of the bacteria are very good and vitally important to the proper functioning of our bodies.

> So be strong and courageous! Do not be afraid and do not panic before them. For the LORD your God will personally go ahead of you. He will neither fail you nor abandon you.
> —DEUTERONOMY 31:6, NLT

On any given day, at least four hundred different varieties of bacteria live and breed in your gastrointestinal tract. That means that approximately a hundred trillion individual bacteria are making residence in your GI tract.

These are the good guys. They form two different types:

- Lactobacillus acidophilus
- Bifido bacteria

These friendly bacteria live in your small and large intestines all the time, controlling mucus, debris, yeast, parasites and overgrowth of pathogenic (bad) bacteria. They also produce vitamin K and B vitamins, and they maintain the proper pH for the digestive tract.

However, if this healthy population of good bacteria is destroyed or reduced in number, your immune system and liver are forced to work much harder to deal with all the impurities and microorganisms that enter into the blood.

Friendly bacteria also neutralize toxins and cancer-causing chemicals and prevent their absorption back into the bloodstream. Good bacteria produce lactic acid, which inhibits the growth of harmful bacteria such as salmonella, shigella and E. coli. These good bacteria also produce fatty acids that make it difficult for candida to survive.

If your body gets overloaded with harmful bacteria you will suffer many different symptoms. Bad bacteria cause foul-smelling stools and painful gas, bloating and abdominal cramps, constipation and diarrhea. Good bacteria, on the other hand, stop bad bacteria from growing and relieve painful gas, constipation and diarrhea.

Good bacteria coat the lining of the intestines, forming a protective barrier against invasions by yeast and other microorganisms.

Lactobacillus acidophilus

Lactobacillus acidophilus is powerful against the growth of candida. This good form of bacteria lives in your small intestines all the time. Lactobacillus bifidus lives mainly in your large intestines.

You can be sure that your body has enough of these important bacteria by drinking lactose-free kefir or by eating lactose-, fruit- and sugar-free yogurt as previously mentioned. During a severe attack of candida overgrowth, you can also choose to supplement with good bacteria.

The DDS-1 strain of lactobacillus acidophilus is a super-efficient strain of acidophilus, which is superior in its ability to attach to the lining of the small intestines and help control yeast overgrowth. DDS-1 is a supplement that can be found in most health food stores. It is important to keep it refrigerated. Take 1 teaspoon two to three times a day.

FOS

FOS (otherwise known as fructooligosaccharides) is a special polysaccharide that is not digested by man, yet feeds friendly bacteria and helps them to grow, while at the same time reducing bad bacteria.

Take 2000 milligrams of FOS a day in order to nourish the good bacteria. You can find FOS at any health food store. It is commonly combined with the acidophilus and bifidus supplements.

> "For I will restore you to health and I will heal you of your wounds," declares the LORD.
>
> —JEREMIAH 30:17, NASB

You should take at least three to five billion organisms of acidophilus and bifidus bacteria on a daily basis in order to recolonize the GI tract. This will enable your body to overcome yeast. This is approximately 1 teaspoon of acidophilus/bifidus two times a day. This should also contain FOS. I recommend BioDophilus-FOS from Biotics, which contains DDS-1 acidophilus, bifidus bacteria and FOS in the recommended dosage.

HEALING YOUR GUT

Candida overgrowth is war that takes place in your gut. Yeast may damage and may even partially destroy the lining of the gastrointestinal tract. That's why it is very important to help your body to heal this war zone.

To heal the lining of the GI tract, I recommend the following supplements:

- L-glutamine, ½–1 tsp. three times a day
- N-acetyl glucosamine, 500 mg. three times a day
- Gamma oryzanol, which is found in rice bran, 300 mg. daily
- FOS, 2000 mg. daily
- Colostrum, one to two 500-mg. capsules three times a day

These supplements can be purchased from a health food store or from a nutritionist.

Two products that I use contain most of these supplements. They are IPS from Biotics and Total Leaky Gut from Nutri-West. I recommend one to two tablets of each three times a day thirty minutes before meals. These are commonly recommended by nutritionists and nutritional doctors.

SUPPLEMENTS TO STRENGTHEN IMMUNITY

Your body's immune system is your first line of defense against the ravages of a yeast attack. Therefore, it's vitally important to strengthen your immune system as much as possible. Here are some important vitamins that will arm your body to wage war against yeast overgrowth.

Sending your immune system to battle against candida overgrowth without giving it vital nutrients and minerals is like sending an army to war without guns. If your body is lacking B_5, B_6, B_{12}, folic acid, vitamin C, vitamin E, vitamin A, selenium, zinc and essential fatty acids, as well as protein, you could be in trouble. It's important to supply your body with the equipment it needs.

Lack of sleep also impairs immune function. Medications such as corticosteroids and antibiotics may deplete the body of B vitamins and zinc, thus impairing immune function. Alcohol and cigarette smoke also impair the immune system.

To be sure that your immune system has the equipment it needs to do its job, here are some important supplements you need to battle candidiasis.

A good multivitamin/multimineral supplement

A deficiency of certain nutrients is probably the most common cause for a poorly functioning immune system. Most Americans are deficient in at least one nutrient. Since a deficiency in any nutrient can result in decreased function of the immune system, it is critically important to take a comprehensive multivitamin and mineral supplement on a daily basis. I recommend Divine Health Multivitamins.

The thymus is a major player in the functioning of your immune system. It orchestrates the working of your immune system throughout your life. When you are born, this gland is larger than your heart. But as you age it gets increasingly smaller. This reduction in size directly corresponds to your immune system's ability to produce disease-fighting T-cells.

Several nutrients can actually prevent this thymus shrinkage. They include:

- Vitamin C
- Vitamin E
- Beta carotene
- Selenium
- Zinc

Vitamin B_6, zinc and vitamin C are needed to improve thymic hormone function.

You can find these nutrients in a comprehensive multivitamin and mineral supplement such as Divine Health Multivitamins.

Zinc

The most important of these supplements for improving thymus function is zinc. When your thymus lacks zinc, vital T-cells are decreased. Take 20–30 milligrams of zinc per day.

Vitamin C

Taking extra doses of vitamin C is extremely important for improving immune function since T-cells contain high levels of vitamin C. Additionally, everyday stress robs your bodies of vitamin C. Therefore, supplementing vitamin C daily is vital for improving your immune system.

I recommend taking high doses of vitamin C daily, approximately 500–1000 milligrams three times a day. However, it is best to take a buffered form of vitamin C.

CONCLUSION

The impact of candida is complicated. It ravages vital organs and robs your body of strength and health until it leaves you feeling completely depleted. But thank goodness that is not the end. With the help of this balanced, well-tested regimen of vitamins, minerals, antioxidants, herbs and other supplements, total restoration for your body is not far away.

> But as for me, I will watch expectantly for the LORD; I will wait for the God of my salvation.
>
> —MICAH 7:7, NASB

But never forget, a doctor can give you a prescription or bind a wound, but only the Great Physician can heal you. Christ is the healer. And regardless of whether you receive a supernatural touch from God or a natural system of vitamins and healthy advice, all healing ultimately comes from Him.

A **BIBLE CURE** Prayer for You

Dear Lord, thank You for providing natural supplements to help restore my body to the perfect balance You planned for it. Thank You for strengthening my body and renewing it from the ravages of candida. Most of all, I thank You for being my healer. Release Your power into my body to free it from the power of sickness and disease. Restore my health and my strength so that I can serve You better. Amen.

A **BIBLE CURE** *Prescription*

Circle the supplements for candida you are planning to take.

Garlic	Goldenseal
Grapefruit extract	Caprylic acid
Oil of oregano	Tanalbit
Chlorophyll supplements	

Circle the medications you plan to discuss with your doctor.

Nystatin   Diflucan

What measures do you plan to take to help your body eliminate dead yeast cell particles and toxins? (circle)

Fiber supplements   Plenty of water

How do you plan to help your body restore good bacteria? (Check the boxes.)

- ❏ Drink sugar-free and lactose-free kefir, 6–8 ounces a day on an empty stomach
- ❏ Eat yogurt that does not contain sugar, lactose or fruit, 6–8 ounces a day
- ❏ Take FOS, DDS-1 acidophilus and bifidus bacteria

What supplements will you take to strengthen immunity? (Check the boxes.)

- ❏ A comprehensive multivitamin/multimineral such as Divine Health Multivitamin
- ❏ A comprehensive antioxidant such as Divine Health Antioxidants
- ❏ Chlorophyll drink such as Divine Health Green Superfood

What supplements will you take to restore your liver? (circle)

Milk thistle	NAC (N-acetyl cysteine)
Taurine	Lipoic acid

Chapter 26

RECOVER YOUR EDGE WITH
LIFESTYLE CHANGES

A LONG TIME AGO a king named David experienced a defeat. He and all his people were robbed. Their goods were taken, their wives and children were taken hostage and their city was burned with fire. When David arrived at the scene and realized what his enemies had done, he responded by praying. He asked God, "'Should I chase after this band of raiders? Will I catch them?' And the LORD told him, 'Yes, go after them. You will surely recover everything that was taken from you!'" (1 Sam. 30:8, NLT).

In a different kind of way, you may be feeling just as David felt when he came back to his city. Perhaps candida has robbed you of your strength, stolen your health and devastated your body. If so, I suggest you do as David did. Go to God and ask Him for help. As with David, He will help you to recover all that your enemy has robbed from you.

> Is there no medicine in Gilead? Is there no physician there?
> Why is there no healing for the wounds of my people?
> —JEREMIAH 8:22, NLT

You know, there were times in the Bible when the Israelites didn't have to fight their enemies. God did it for them and they just watched. But other times they had to go out and fight the battle with God's help. They never regarded one victory as being more from God than the other. They believed God's help was with them in each situation.

Healing is just like that. Sometimes God simply touches a body supernaturally and a person is healed. I've witnessed many such moments of divine intervention. Still, there are other times when God tells us to go and fight our physical battle. But whether we are healed in a sparkling supernatural moment or we go into battle, God's promise is with us as it was with David. He says, "Go, for you will recover all."

This Bible Cure book is providing you with weapons for your battle, powerful keys that with God's help will ensure your success. So let's look at another key: lifestyle changes that can give you an edge in your battle.

Do You Get Enough Rest?

Your immune system is dependent upon the rest you give it. If you burn your candle at both ends, eventually the ends will meet at the middle and your immune system will become depleted.

To strengthen your immune system so that it can effectively battle candida, you must sleep at least eight hours at night. Getting enough rest is important all the time, but it's especially important during the battle you're in.

Minimizing Stress

Stress drains your immune system as little else does. Therefore, support your body's fight against yeast by minimizing as much stress in your life as possible.

Here are some pointers:

- Don't work extra hours while your body is battling yeast.
- Don't take on any new projects or new obligations.
- Simplify your life as much as possible until you are well. Learn how to rest, conserve, preserve and rebuild your immune system.

Mercury, a Hidden Enemy

One thing you may not have thought of in your battle against candida is your teeth. If your mouth is full of old amalgam fillings, you may have a hidden enemy.

Your immune system could be suppressed by mercury toxicity, which is usually due to amalgam fillings in the teeth. These are actually silver fillings. Silver fillings are primarily composed of silver, mercury and tin. The mercury contained in these silver fillings is very dangerous to the human body.

If you have silver fillings, then you probably have an overgrowth of candida in your GI tract. Hundreds of published scientific papers directly link the mercury released from these amalgam fillings to chronic disease.

If you have these fillings, mercury is continually being released in your mouth. Every time you brush your teeth, chew gum or drink hot beverages, mercury vapor is released, increasing the release of mercury. In fact, those with amalgam fillings or silver fillings have an average mercury vapor content that's ten times higher than those without silver fillings. About 80 percent of this inhaled mercury vapor is then actually absorbed into your bloodstream.

The mercury that is released in your body binds to the mineral receptor sites for zinc, selenium and other minerals, thus further depressing your immune system.

To speak with a well-informed nutritional doctor who knows how to diagnose and treat mercury toxicity, call 1-800-LEADOUT to find a doctor near you. To find a biological dentist, call GLCCM at (800) 286-6013. If your dentist is not trained in the proper removal of mercury, please call GLCCM and find one who is. Improper removal of silver fillings can seriously impair the immune system, impeding your recovery from candida.

CONCLUSION

If you have discovered that enemies of toxins and stress have attacked you body even more than you realized, don't be alarmed. Do what David did—look to God for help. God promises never to fail you nor forsake you. The Bible says, "Be strong and courageous, do not be afraid or tremble at them, for the LORD your God is the one who goes with you. He will not fail you or forsake you" (Deut. 31:6, NASB).

With God's help, you will recover all!

A **BIBLE CURE** *Prayer for You*

Dear God, thank You that You promise total recovery of health and strength to my body. Thank You that You promise to never fail me or leave me no matter what I am battling or going through. Your love and care for my life mean so much to me. I am truly grateful. Help me to make the lifestyle changes neces- sary to battle my enemies of sickness and disease, and most of all, help me to use my good health and vitality to serve You. Amen.

A **BIBLE CURE** *Prescription*

Write a prayer thanking God for His help in recovering all.

_____

_____

_____

_____

_____

List the things in your life that you want God to help you recover.

_____

_____

_____

_____

_____

_____

Chapter 27

RECHARGE YOUR
SPIRIT WITH FAITH

U NTIL NOW WE'VE looked at many natural things you can do to recover the good health that God intended for you. Let's take a moment to look at the energizing power of faith.

Faith recharges your spirit, giving you the power to reach beyond this material world and take hold of the healing power of God. Hear what the Bible says about faith: "And this is the victory that overcomes the world—our faith" (1 John 5:4, NKJV).

The final key in your Bible cure is the power of faith. This transcendent force has overcome kingdoms and risen above every obstacle.

Depression and stress are perhaps two of the worst things that can happen to your immune system. Both of them can do amazing damage to your body and tremendously impair its ability to function. When you are depressed, your immune system tends to be depressed as well. When you are stressed out, your immune system is stressed, too.

The amount of immune suppression is usually related to the amount of stress you are under. During periods of stress people are far more prone to infection because of the lowered immune function caused by stress.

TAKE FIVE

The energizing power of faith will form a mighty shield against the destructive power of stress and depression. Here are five ways to arm yourself.

Take time to relax.

Your body will enter into a deep state of relaxation when you praise and worship God and meditate on the Word of God. Deep-breathing exercises, massages and even taking a hot bath while playing soothing worship music will also greatly relax your body. Praise and worship music gets into your spirit, and the peace it gives provides an internal shield against stress, depression and anxiety.

Get to know your body. Take note of when you feel particularly stressed out and what changes take place. After a particularly stressful day or event, give special attention to relaxing your body and your nerves. A few moments of relaxation will allow your immune system to recover from the damaging effects of stress.

Take a moment to laugh.

Most people battling candida overgrowth are stressed out and depressed. Therefore, they usually have a very low-functioning immune system. Their cortisol and adrenaline levels are usually either elevated or extremely depressed. The best medicine for overcoming stress and depression is laughter. In fact, the Bible says that a merry heart does good like a medicine. (See Proverbs 17:22.)

Norman Cousins wrote the book *Anatomy of an Illness As Perceived by the Patient* in 1979.[1] Cousins used laughter to fight a serious disease, actually laughing his way back to health. He watched funny movies such as the Marx Brothers films. He watched funny TV shows such as *Candid Camera* and read funny books.

A good belly laugh is able to stimulate all the major organs like a massage. Laughter also helps to raise your energy level and helps to pull you out of the pit of depression. Take at least a ten- to twenty-minute laughter break a day. Watch funny movies and TV shows. Read jokes in the newspaper, books or magazines, and share these clean jokes with others because laughter is contagious. Instead of looking critically at a situation, find out what's funny about it.

Joy gives you strength. The Bible says, "Don't be dejected and sad, for the joy of the Lord is your strength!" (Neh. 8:10).

> Restore to me the joy of your salvation, and make me willing
> to obey you.
>
> —PSALM 51:12, NLT

You may be thinking, *That's easy for him to say. He doesn't know my circumstances!* No one but God truly knows another's circumstances, thoughts and feelings. But that doesn't matter; you can find joy, not in circumstances, but in Christ. The Bible promises, "You will make known to me the path of life; in Your presence is fulness of joy; in Your right hand there are pleasures forever" (Ps. 16:11, NASB).

I encourage you to find joy in life by knowing Christ.

The average man and woman laughs about four to eight times a day. The average child laughs about 150 times a day. Strengthen your immune system by beginning to laugh more today.

Take refuge in the Scriptures.

God's Word breaks the destructive power of certain deadly emotions such as fear, rage, hatred, resentment, bitterness, shame and so forth. I encourage you to quote scriptures related to them at least three times a day on a continuous basis. Also consider reading and meditating on Bible passages like 1 Corinthians 13, the chapter on love, since there is no greater force in the universe than the power of God's love. It is able to break the bondage of any destructive emotion.

Take up positive attitudes.

Related to Scripture reading is the practice of "putting on" the positive, healthy emotions that it speaks of—emotions like love, joy, peace, patience, kindness, goodness and self-control. We know that certain emotions are associated with lowered immune function and higher cortisol levels. Approaching life with the biblical "attitude prescription" will help you avoid the damaging effects of stress, fear and worry.

A **BIBLE CURE** *Prayer for You*

Dear Jesus Christ, thank You for dying on the cross to pay the cost of mankind's sins, including my own. I give You all my sins and repent for each and every one. I ask You to come into my heart and life. And I surrender myself and my future to Your will and to Your care. Thank You for suffering under the Roman lash so that I can be healed and made completely whole. I receive You right now. In Jesus' name, amen.

A **BIBLE CURE** *Prescription*

Faith Builder

He was pierced through for our transgressions, He was crushed for our iniquities; the chastening for our well-being fell upon Him, and by His scourging we are healed.

—ISAIAH 53:5, NASB

Read this dynamic scripture several times aloud. It has great power! Insert your own name into it.

He was pierced through for _____ transgressions, He was crushed for _____ iniquities; the chastening of _____ well-being fell upon Him, and by His scourging _____ is healed!

THE BIBLE

CURE

RECIPES FOR
OVERCOMING
CANDIDA

Chapter 28

RESTORING YOUR HEALTH
WITH NUTRITION

G OD IS IN the business of restoring His people to health! He promises this in His Word: "'I will give you back your health and heal your wounds,' says the LORD" (Jer. 30:17, NLT). His desire is to renew and restore you—body, soul, mind and spirit. The Bible says, "Dear friend, I hope all is well with you and that you are as healthy in body as you are strong in spirit" (3 John 2, NLT).

Many individuals have healthy souls, but they are living their lives here on earth in sick or weakened bodies. Perhaps you have been weakened or made ill by the effects of candida (yeast) running rampant in your body. If so, take heart! God has provided a way out for you! The most powerful way to combat the effects of yeast imbalances in your body is through the practice of sound, healthy nutritional habits.

In *The Bible Cure for Candida and Yeast Infections*, I explain the nutritional habits that will help cure these conditions. And in this Bible Cure book, you will discover healthy, nutritious and delicious recipes to help you develop these good nutritional habits. First, I will introduce the basic facts regarding candida to help you make healthy changes in your eating habits.

WHAT IS CANDIDA?

Candida, or the yeast syndrome, is simply an overgrowth of yeast that usually lives in the intestinal tract. But in women it can also manifest in painful infections in the vagina. When yeast overgrows in the GI tract, it can cause a number of distressing symptoms, including heartburn, indigestion, abdominal bloating, cramps, constipation or diarrhea, nausea or gas.

Are you experiencing these symptoms? If so, you may be exhibiting signs of an overgrowth of candida. I suggest that you also read *The Bible Cure Book for Candida and Yeast Infections.* It contains further descriptions of this problem as well as dietary and supplement information that will help you restore balance in your intestinal tract and health throughout your body.

Everyone has various kinds of yeast living on his or her skin and in the intestinal tract. Candida, one type of yeast found within the human intestines, is quite normal and is compatible with a lifetime of excellent health. Its growth is generally held in check by the presence of "good" bacteria also present in the intestines. However, under the influence of various medications, dietary choices and stress, the delicate balance between the good bacteria and candida can become disrupted. Then the once harmless levels of yeast grow out of control and may begin to invade and colonize throughout the body.

This Bible Cure book is filled with nutritional facts, delicious recipes and cooking tips to help you overcome candida. But even more importantly, it will encourage you to stand strong against temptation by the power of God's Word and begin to apply godly principles to your eating habits. In this book, you will

> *uncover God's divine plan of health for body, soul and*
> *spirit through modern medicine, good nutrition and*
> *the medicinal power of Scripture and prayer.*

You will also discover life-changing scriptures throughout this book that will strengthen and encourage you.

As you read and choose to apply and trust God's promises, it will help you to use the powerful Bible Cure prayers I have included to line up your thoughts and feelings with God's plan of divine health for you, a plan that includes living victoriously.

It is my prayer that these recipes and nutritional tips will help restore wholeness to your life—spirit, soul and body. And may this book also deepen your fellowship with God and strengthen your ability to worship and serve Him.

A **BIBLE CURE** *Prayer for You*

Lord, I thank You that You desire to restore me to health: spirit, soul and body! Please teach me the things I need to change in my diet and nutritional habits to overcome the overgrowth of candida in my body, and give me strength to apply these principles in my life. In Jesus' name, amen.

Chapter 29

BE AN OVERCOMER!

F YOU HAVE been held captive by the weakening effects of candida overgrowth in your body, it is important for you to realize that *this problem can be overcome!* God is on your side, ready to help. If you turn to Him, He will empower you with the strength you need to be an overcomer in this area of your life.

The Bible tells us that "he gives power to those the weak and strength to the powerless. Even youths will become weak and tired, and young men will fall in exhaustion. But those who trust in the LORD will find new strength. They will soar high on wings like eagles. They will run and not grow weary. They will walk and not faint" (Isa. 40:29–31, NLT).

> I am the LORD who heals you.
>
> —EXODUS 15:26, NLT

If you are ready and willing to make a change in your life, this Bible Cure book is for you. Rely on God's strength to help you implement the nutritional changes you need to make in your diet—and to follow through with those changes.

First, let's consider briefly the causes and symptoms of this problem—as well as the role that nutrition can play in alleviating it.

CAUSES AND SYMPTOMS

The overgrowth of candida is prevented by "good" bacteria, which are usually present in our colon. However, antibiotics, certain environmental factors, as well as bad nutritional habits, can deplete the amount of good bacteria that are actively working on our behalf.

When this occurs, candida begins to grow out of control in the intestinal tract, producing mycotoxins, which are toxins produced by yeast, and potentially causing many serious problems. This yeast overgrowth syndrome is known as *candidiasis*.

Diverse causes

Factors that trigger candidiasis include using antibiotics, birth control pills and corticosteroids prescribed for treatment of disease. Another trigger is eating sugar and highly processed carbohydrates.

Yeast multiplies rapidly in the body by feeding on sugar. The average American consumes 150 pounds of sugar per year. In many cases, that is more than a person's own body weight! When you decide to indulge in desserts such as cakes, pies, cookies, brownies and the like, you are literally inviting the candida in your body to a feast!

> You must serve only the LORD your God. If you do, I will bless you with food and water, and I will protect you from illness.
> —EXODUS 23:25, NLT

Distressing symptoms

Yeast overgrowth is able to produce seventy-nine known toxins. One of the most toxic substances produced by yeast is acetaldehyde. When this substance enters into the liver, it is converted into alcohol. Acetaldehyde contributes to a raft of harmful symptoms, including fatigue, mental cloudiness, disorientation, confusion, irritability, headaches, anxiety and depression.

Not only does yeast overgrowth produce these distressing symptoms, but it also depletes minerals, it increases free radical formation, and it disrupts enzymes the body needs to produce energy.

If the yeast overgrowth continues unchecked, it can further weaken our immune system, and its mycotoxins may then affect any organ or tissue in the body. As soon as a particular organ in your body is affected, symptoms flair. For instance, as candida or its toxic waste products affect the nervous system, you may begin to experience fatigue, memory loss, insomnia, depression, mood swings, sleepiness, attention-deficit disorder, hyperactivity, or autistic tendencies.

Many diseases and illnesses are usually yeast related, including those listed below:

A **BIBLE CURE** Health Fact

Yeast-Related Diseases and Illnesses

- Chronic fatigue syndrome
- Severe allergies
- Multiple chemical sensitivities
- Endometriosis
- Infertility
- Decreased sex drive
- Eczema
- Rheumatoid arthritis
- Multiple sclerosis
- Recurrent ear infections
- Bronchitis
- Sinusitis

- Attention-deficit hyperactivity disorder
- Food allergies
- Premenstrual syndrome
- Interstitial cystitis
- Sexual dysfunction
- Psoriasis
- Asthma
- Lupus
- Autism
- Most autoimmune disorders
- Fibromyalgia

From the diseases and illnesses listed, you can see that when yeast grows out of control it can weaken the body, wreaking havoc wherever it goes. And the toxins produced by candida can make you feel absolutely miserable.

If you suspect you may be suffering from yeast overgrowth, take the self-test on page 292 to see how you stack up.

THE ROLE OF NUTRITION

When I discuss the possibility of candida overgrowth with my patients, I usually ask them one very important question: "What foods do you crave?" Most patients with a candida problem have one answer in common: "I crave sugar!"

If you are a person who can't resist cakes, pies, cookies, colas, chocolate, breads, ice cream, alcohol or other processed foods that are high in sugar and carbohydrates, it is time to take control of your eating habits! You are literally feeding the problem. Even some foods that are considered to be healthy, like fruits and fruit juices, can contribute to an overgrowth of yeast in the body.

> I have heard your prayer and seen your tears. I will heal you.
> —2 Kings 20:5, NLT

Fortunately, there is a way to eat healthy foods that are high in nutritional content, which will decrease the growth of candida—and they are delicious as well! Keep reading to discover the specially-formulated recipes and nutritional tips designed specifically to reduce candida and put you back on track to a balanced lifestyle and a strong, healthy body.

 A **BIBLE CURE** *Prescription*

Are there any foods that you crave? If so, what are they?

_____

_____

_____

_____

Are you willing to make necessary changes in your diet to combat candida overgrowth in your body? If so, pray the following prayer:

Heavenly Father, Your Word says that You will restore my body to health and give me a long, satisfied life. I stand on Your promises today as I begin to confront this problem of candida overgrowth in my body. Thank You for Your wisdom that will show me the specific steps I need to take to walk in health. In Jesus' name I pray. Amen.

Chapter 30

LAYING THE GROUND RULES

Overcoming candida will require you to stay on the candida diet for a period of time. Yet the world we live in constantly barrages us with advertisements for "fast foods," sugar-filled, and highly processed foods. But while discipline must play a key role in maintaining this diet, the good news is that your meals do not have to be boring and dull!

> O Lord my God, I cried to you for help, and you restored my health.
>
> —Psalm 30:2, NLT

The Bible says, "The joy of the Lord is your strength!" (Neh. 8:10, NLT); it also tells us to "go ahead. Eat your food with joy, and drink your wine with a happy heart, for God approves of this!" (Eccles. 9:7, NLT). How can anyone eat their food with a happy heart if their meal is boring, bland or monotonous—if they are following a diet out of drudgery? This book will provide you with simple, delicious recipes that will make it a joy to follow the candida diet.

To begin, we need to establish the following guidelines for a few weeks to ensure your success. If this list of *nos* seems overwhelming to you, let me remind you of the delicious recipes that are waiting for you to try in the next chapters. For now, commit to the following:

1. No sugar of any kind may be consumed on this diet. That includes white sugar, brown sugar, honey, molasses, syrup, sucrose, lactose, maltose, fructose or corn syrup.

2. No artificial sweeteners are allowed, including Sweet 'N Low, NutraSweet or Equal. However, Stevia and Splenda are acceptable.

3. No fruit juice is allowed. After the candida is brought under control, a small amount of grapefruit juice may be permitted.

4. No fruit of any kind may be consumed during the first three weeks of the diet. After the third week, some low-sugar fruits may gradually be introduced, such as apples, pears, kiwis, blueberries, blackberries, raspberries, strawberries, grapefruit, lemons and limes.

5. No lactose is allowed; therefore, no milk, cheese, cottage cheese, ice cream or sour cream is permitted. A small amount of organic butter and yogurt or kefir may be used, as long as it contains no lactose, sugar or fruit.

6. No gluten grains may be eaten. These include wheat, rye, white or pumpernickel breads, as well as pastries, pasta, crackers, etc. Oat products usually contain less gluten and may be eaten by those with less severe candida overgrowth. Grains that are acceptable include brown rice bread or crackers; millet bread; spelt bread, crackers or pasta; and brown rice.

7. No foods containing yeast of any kind are permitted—including bakery products or commercially prepared food products.

8. No alcoholic beverages of any kind may be consumed.

9. No dry roasted nuts are allowed. However, nuts in the shell—other than peanuts, pistachios or cashews—are acceptable, because the shell keeps these nuts from molding.

10. No vinegar or vinegar-containing foods are allowed. (The possible exception would be raw unfiltered apple cider vinegar only for those with mild cases of candida.)

11. No soy sauce, tamari or natural root beer is allowed.

12. No vitamin or mineral supplements containing yeast may be taken.

13. No pickled foods or smoked, dried or cured meats, including bacon, may be eaten. This includes processed lunchmeats, sausage, hot dogs, salami, bologna, etc.

14. No deep-fried foods of any kind are allowed.

15. No mushrooms may be eaten.

16. No caffeinated beverages may be consumed, including coffee, teas and sodas. Instead, choose herbal teas, such as dandelion root tea, pau d'arco, fruit teas or mint tea, but be sure they do not contain citric acid.

17. No corn of any kind may be eaten, including corn on the cob, corn chips, popcorn, corn meal, etc.

18. No refined oils may be used in cooking, including sunflower oil, safflower oil or corn oil. Instead, use cold-pressed oils such as extra-virgin olive oil.

19. Avoid potatoes and sweet potatoes since these are rapidly converted to sugars within the body.

Although these ground rules may seem intimidating at first, if you persevere with these dietary changes, the results in your health and overall energy levels will be dramatic. After about three months of avoiding these foods, many candida patients find that they can gradually re-introduce some of them into their diet, rotating them every three to four days. But some foods should always be avoided for those with a candida problem, including foods that are high in sugar such as sugary desserts, ice cream and alcoholic beverages.

A **BIBLE CURE** Health Fact

On the nutritional labels of food products, most sugars are the substances that end with the letters "o-s-e."

STRENGTHENING THE IMMUNE SYSTEM

As your immune system grows weaker, the candida in your body has the opportunity to grow stronger. As you begin to follow the candida diet to restore your body to health, it is important to not forget these crucial steps to strengthen your immune system.

- Be sure to get eight to ten hours of sleep each night.
- Take a Sabbath day of rest each week.
- Decrease your stress.
- Take steps to simplify your life.
- Practice having a merry heart!

> The LORD nurses them when they are sick and restores them to health.
>
> —PSALM 41:3, NLT

SUPPLEMENTS CAN HELP

In addition to getting sufficient rest and reducing your stress levels, it may be helpful to take nutritional supplements to modulate your immune system. Moducare and Natur-Leaf are plant sterols and ste-rolins, which are helpful for this condition. I recommend taking either Moducare or Natur-Leaf. Moducare is found at most health food stores; the recommended dosage is two capsules in the morning and one in the evening on an empty stomach. Natur-Leaf must be ordered. (See appendix B for ordering information.) The recom-mended dosage is one capsule twice a day on an empty stomach or one hour before meals.

Author's note: For more information on any of these supplements or testing procedures mentioned in this section, refer to appendix B at the back of this book.

Total Leaky Gut

In addition to supplements that bring balance to the immune system, it can also be helpful to take other nutritional supplements while on the candida diet. To heal damage done to the GI tract, I recommend taking Total Leaky Gut at a dose of one tablet, three times a day, thirty minutes before meals.

Beneficial bacteria

To overcome candida, it is critically important to restore beneficial bacteria to the GI tract. To do this, I recommend multiple forms of beneficial bacterial, including Divine Health Probiotic at a dose of two tablets twice a day on an empty stomach. Three Lac is another excellent probiotic; I recommend one packet twice a day before meals. Finally, Probiotic Pearls, one tablet twice daily, is also important.

> Lord, your discipline is good, for it leads to life and health. You restore my health and allow me to live!
>
> —Isaiah 38:16, NLT

Antifungal agents

In addition, an antifungal agent should be taken to reduce the yeast levels in the intestinal tract. For patients with a mild candida problem, I recommend Divine Health Candida Formula, in a dosage of one tablet three times a day.

Some patients may need something stronger, such as Nystatin, which must be prescribed by a physician.

Other patients are so infested with yeast that they need an even more potent medication such as Diflucan, which must be closely monitored by a doctor.

Biotin

To keep candida in its noninvasive form, most candida patients need to take a supplement of biotin, at a dose of 1,000-microgram capsule three times a day. This nutrient is usually deficient in patients with candidiasis. Biotin may be found in most health food stores.

Help for allergies

Most candida patients have numerous food allergies or sensitivities, and an excellent way to desensitize them is with NAET, a noninvasive, drug-free, natural solution to treat allergies of all types. Their Web site is www.naet.com

You can also determine your food allergies with a blood test such as the ALCAT test. (See appendix B.)

A **BIBLE CURE** *Health Tip*

There may be times when avoiding sugar is impossible. A birthday party, holiday seasons or other celebrations may make it very difficult to pass up foods that you would not ordinarily eat. On those occasions, remember to exercise self-control and take an extra biotin supplement and a natural anti-fungal agent, such as Divine Health Candida Formula, to counteract the sugars in your system.

MORE FACTORS TO CONSIDER

Most candida patients can restore health simply by following the candida diet and taking the supplements listed above. However, if after six months your symptoms have still not improved, you should consider the possibility of other contributing factors to your condition. Some of these factors may include the following:

1. *A hormone imbalance.* There may be adrenal, thyroid or sex hormone imbalance present. Many patients with candida suffer from subclinical hypothyroidism and should take a natural thyroid supplement. Most candida patients also have low adrenal function and require an adrenal supplement such as DSF, one tablet two times a day. (See appendix B.) Women may need natural progesterone cream, which can be obtained from a health food store, and men may need natural testosterone cream, which must be prescribed by a physician and can be compounded at a compounding pharmacy. Call Pharmacy Specialists at 1-407-260-7002 to find a physician in your area.

2. *An untreated parasitic, viral or bacterial infection*

3. *A toxic heavy metal*—such as mercury, lead or cadmium—in your system.

4. *Emotional problems* such as frustration, unforgiveness, guilt, rejection, depression or anxiety.

5. *A nutritional deficiency.* Because most candida patients cannot take a multivitamin initially in their treatment, this problem may need to be addressed after other issues, such as food allergies or sensitivities, are resolved.

6. *A digestion problem.* Many candida patients have poor digestion and may need to take a digestive enzyme or a hydrochloric acid supplement. However, just as with many other supplements, this should be introduced after the initial problems are resolved.

7. *Acidosis.* Acidosis is a condition in which body tissues become overly acidic, as indicated by a urine pH test. Acidosis in the body promotes the growth of candida. For these patients, I recommend Vaxa's Buffer pH, one tablet three times a day.

8. *Excessive amounts of stress*

A **BIBLE CURE** Health Tip

The Bible says that "a cheerful heart is good medicine, but a broken spirit saps a person's strength" (Prov. 17:22, NLT). It is a scientific fact that laughing is good for you; it releases endorphins and reduces stress levels. I recommend ten belly laughs a day in order to stimulate the immune system.

Why not go out and purchase a joke book or watch a funny movie? Learn to laugh a little more. Before you know it, everything will stop seeming so serious.

HOW LONG SHOULD I STAY ON THE DIET?

The candida diet is foundational to any good candida program. This strict diet is required for a sufficient period of time to reduce yeast overgrowth. Withholding foods on which it thrives will weaken it and allow the good bacteria to regain their important balance. The period of time varies from individual to individual due to the strength of their immune system and the severity of the disease that is being manifested.

> Your salvation will come like the dawn, and your wounds will quickly heal.
>
> —ISAIAH 58:8, NLT

If you have chronic fatigue or fibromyalgia, you may need to follow the candida diet for six months to a year. If you are experiencing an autoimmune disorder, you may need to be on the program for one or two years. If you are experiencing less serious symptoms of PMS, fatigue, cloudy thinking, and muscle and joint aches and pains, you may only need to be on the program three to six months.

Everyone is different, and there are a number of factors involved in determining the length of time you should stay on the candida diet. These factors include:

- The severity of the yeast overgrowth
- The strength of your immune system
- The degree of your food sensitivities
- The severity of the disease

This program involves three phases. Phase 1 is the first twenty-one days and is used to detoxify the body, break any food addictions and begin to eliminate food sensitivities. Phase 2 is an excellent program to bring candida under control, eliminate food allergies and enable you to lose weight. Phase 3 is the stabilization stage where your symptoms of candida have resolved or you have achieved your goal weight and your food sensitivities are under control. In phase 3 you can eat almost anything with the exception of foods high in sugar, highly processed foods and any other foods to which you are still sensitive or allergic.

Phase 1—the first three weeks

You will eat no sugar of any kind, including fruits. Also, avoid completely wheat, corn, dairy (except for a small amount of organic butter), artificial flavorings, sweeteners, food additives, yeast, vinegar, soy sauce, pickled foods, smoked or cured meats, potatoes, mushrooms, deep-fried foods, and gluten grains (such as wheat products).

Phase 2

You can add low-glycemic fruits back to your diet, such as Granny Smith apples, berries (blueberries, blackberries, raspberries, strawberries), grapefruit and kiwi. You can add all veggies except white potatoes and corn. You may be able to add oats back to your diet. See pages 282–284 for foods to avoid.

Phase 3

Add everything back to your diet except foods high in sugar and highly processed foods, as well as any foods to which you are still sensitive.

I recommend that everyone who starts the candida diet remain under the care of a good nutritional doctor who can monitor your progress. Many conventional medical doctors do not recognize candida or candida-related illnesses.

> Let all that I am praise the LORD....He forgives all my sins and heals all my diseases.
> —PSALM 103:2–3, NLT

ENJOYING DELICIOUS HELP

In the following chapters of this book you will find many delicious recipes that will assist you in following the candida diet. Instead of indulging in that chocolate chip cookie or piece of lemon meringue pie, you can enjoy healthy, nutritious foods—and desserts, too—that are not only delicious, but will help restore your body to the divine health that God has for you!

A **BIBLE CURE** *Prayer for You*

Dear Lord, I realize that You have created my body and that You know what is best for it. I ask You for the self-control I need to maintain the nutritional guidelines I know are healthy for me and that will restore my body to a normal balance and level of functioning. Holy Spirit, help me control what I eat. Help reduce my cravings for sugar, for desserts that I should not have, and increase my desire for the foods that I should eat. Give me discipline to do the things You ask me to do so that I can walk in health all the days of my life. In Jesus' name, amen.

A **BIBLE CURE** Prescription

Would you like to know how much of your health problem is yeast related? If so, then take the candida quiz below and add up your points to see how you stack up.[1]

1. Have you taken tetracycline or other antibiotics for acne for one month or longer?   (25 points) _____

2. Have you ever taken other broad-spectrum antibiotics for respiratory, urinary or other infections for two months or longer, or in short courses four or more times in one year?   (20 points) _____

3. Have you ever taken a broad-spectrum antibiotic (even a single course)?   (6 points) _____

4. Have you ever been bothered by persistent prostatitis, vaginitis or other problems affecting your reproductive organs?   (25 points) _____

5. Have you been pregnant one time?   (3 points) _____
   Two or more times?   (5 points) _____

6. Have you taken birth control pills?
   For six months to two years?   (8 points) _____
   For more than two years?   (15 points) _____

7. Have you taken prednisone or other cortisone-type drugs?
   For two weeks or less?   (6 points) _____
   For more than two weeks?   (15 points) _____

8. Does exposure to perfumes, insecticides, fabric shop odors or other chemicals provoke:
   Mild symptoms?   (5 points) _____
   Moderate to severe symptoms?   (20 points) _____

9. Are your symptoms worse on damp, muggy days or in moldy places?   (20 points) _____

10. Have you had athlete's foot, ringworm, "jock-itch" or other chronic infections of the skin or nails?
    Mild to moderate?   (10 points) _____
    Severe or persistent?   (20 points) _____

11. Do you crave sugar? (10 points) _____

12. Do you crave breads? (10 points) _____

13. Do you crave alcoholic beverages? (10 points) _____

14. Does tobacco smoke really
bother you? (10 points) _____

How to score the candida quiz

If you are a woman and scored over 180, yeast-connected problems are almost certainly present. If you are a man and scored over 140, yeast-connected problems are almost certainly present.

If you are a woman and scored 120–180, yeast-connected health problems are probably present. If you are a man and scored 90–140, yeast-connected health problems are probably present.

If you are a woman and scored 60–119, yeast-connected health problems are possibly present. If you are a man and scored 40–89, yeast-connected health problems are possibly present.

If you are a woman and scored less than 60, or a man and scored less than 40, yeast-connected health problems are less likely present.

I also commonly perform a blood test to diagnose candida over-growth. The blood test is called *Candida Immune Complexes and Antibodies*. If these tests are elevated, you should definitely begin the candida diet as well as take the supplements. Your physician can order this test by calling AAL Reference Laboratory Inc. at 1-800-552-2611.

Chapter 31

YUMMY BREAKFASTS

CALIFORNIA OMELET[1]

Phase 1, 2, 3

4 large organic eggs (or Egg Beaters)

1 medium avocado, scrubbed, peeled and diced

1 can (2.2-ounce) sliced ripe olives, drained (optional

1 large tomato, scrubbed and diced)

2 Tbsp. clarified butter (found in most health food stores; if you are unable to find, use organic butter)

2 large green onions, scrubbed, peeled and coarsely chopped

Beat eggs in a medium bowl with a rotary beater or electric mixer. Add other ingredients, except butter; mix. Place butter in a large skillet; melt, moving pan back and forth until entire surface and sides are coated. Add egg mixture; cook over medium heat until sides and bottom are golden brown. Turn half of omelet over other half; cover. Cook at low heat until egg is set and omelet is golden brown.

10 grams carbs; serves 2.

SCRAMBLED EGGS FIESTA[2]

Phase 1, 2, 3

6 large organic whole eggs (or Egg Beaters)
½ cup chopped red bell peppers
1 Tbsp. minced jalapeno pepper (about 1)
1 fresh avocado, sliced
4 spelt tortillas
½ cup chopped onion
½ cup chopped green peppers
1 Tbsp. organic butter
1 can Bearitos Vegetarian Refried Black Beans
4 Tbsp. fresh salsa

Heat butter in a sauté pan and add peppers and onions; sauté until slightly soft. Scramble eggs in a separate bowl and add to pan; reduce heat and cook until eggs are scrambled.

Serve with avocado slices, salsa, refried black beans and spelt tortilla.

39 grams carbs; serves 4.

FRITTATA PRIMAVERA[3]

Phase 1, 2, 3

¾ Tbsp. extra-virgin olive oil (or organic butter)
½ cup chopped red bell peppers
½ cup thinly sliced onions
½ cup thinly sliced zucchini
½ cup chopped fresh tomato (liquid drained)
½ tsp. cracked black pepper
6 organic eggs, beaten
1 Tbsp. fresh basil chiffonade
1 Tbsp. fresh parsley, minced
Sea salt to taste

In a large skillet (nonstick is preferable), heat ½ Tbsp. olive oil on medium heat; add chopped red bell peppers and sauté for two minutes. Add sliced onions and sauté for 5 minutes or until soft. Add zucchini and chopped, drained tomatoes, and sauté for 2 minutes. Add cracked pepper and beaten eggs.

As eggs begin to set, loosen sides with a heat-resistant spatula. Continue to cook on medium heat (adjust heat as necessary), and cover to finish cooking the top. When top is cooked, loosen frittata and slide onto serving platter. Cut into serving portions as you would a pie. Sprinkle with sea salt if desired.

4 grams carbs; serves 3.

POACHED EGGS[4]

Phase 1, 2, 3

2 poached organic eggs
2 slices spelt or millet toast
1 tsp. butter

Serves 1.

BLUEBERRY BUCKWHEAT PANCAKES

Phase 2, 3

1 cup buckwheat pancake mix
¾ cup unsweetened soy milk
1 Tbsp. extra-virgin olive oil
1–2 cups blueberries

Heat skillet over medium-low heat.

Combine all ingredients except blueberries and stir with a wire whisk until large lumps disappear. Let stand 1–2 minutes to thicken.

Pour slightly less than ¼ cup for each pancake onto skillet, lightly greased with organic butter or extra-virgin olive oil. Sprinkle blueberries as desired on top of pancakes while cooking. Turn when pancakes bubble and bottoms are golden brown. Use sugar-free syrup made with Stevia, glycerin or sucralose.

23 grams carbs; makes 12–14 pancakes.

MILLET OR RICE CEREAL

Phase 1, 2, 3

Use unsweetened soy, rice or almond milk with millet or rice cereal with no added sugars. You may add berries to your cereal. (This is not phase 1 if you add berries.)

Millet cereal, 77 grams carbs; rice cereal, 29 grams carbs; serves 1.

OLD-FASHIONED OATMEAL

Phase 2, 3

Cook your old-fashioned oatmeal in water or unsweetened soy, rice or almond milk and a small amount of organic butter. Sweeten with Stevia or Splenda. Serve with spelt or millet toast.

Serves 1.

BROWN RICE GRITS[5]

Phase 1, 2, 3

¼ cup dry Arrowhead Mills Rice & Shine
¾ cup water
2 tsp. organic butter, if desired
¼ cup unsweetened soy milk
1 tsp. chopped pecans
¼ tsp. cinnamon
1/16 tsp. Stevia (if extra sweetness is desired)

Add cereal to water and bring to boil, stirring constantly. Reduce heat, cover and simmer for about 2 minutes, until desired consistency is reached. Place in serving bowls and add rest of ingredients as desired to enhance grits.

CAUTION: High in carbohydrates.

6 grams carbs; serves 2.

FRENCH TOAST[6]

Phase 1, 2, 3

3 whole organic eggs

¼ cup unsweetened soy milk

8 slices millet bread

½ tsp. ground nutmeg

½ tsp. ground cinnamon

1 Tbsp. organic butter

In a pie plate, whip eggs until smooth. Add soy milk, nutmeg and cinnamon. Heat butter in a sauté pan over medium heat. Briefly soak slices of bread in egg mixture and cook on both sides until golden brown. Hold on heated platter until ready to serve. Add more butter to pan as necessary. Use sugar-free syrup made with Stevia, glycerin or sucralose.

32 grams carbs; serves 4.

Chapter 32

SIMPLE SALADS

CHICKEN SALAD[1]

Phase 1, 2, 3

2 cups finely chopped cooked chicken
½ cup finely chopped celery
2–4 chopped hard-boiled eggs
1 medium onion, chopped

Moisten with sugar/honey-free mayonnaise, obtainable from your health food store.

4 grams carbs; serves 4.

GRILLED SHRIMP SALAD[2]

Phase 1, 2, 3

1½ lbs. medium to large shrimp, with shell and tail removed
2 Tbsp. olive oil
1 tsp. granulated garlic
1 tsp. cracked black pepper
¼ tsp. sea salt
1 Tbsp. chopped fresh parsley
1 lb. bag of mixed lettuce
1 cup cubed fresh tomatoes

Place raw cleaned shrimp in bowl and add olive oil, garlic, salt, pepper and fresh parsley. Coat shrimp thoroughly, marinate for 10–20 minutes. Heat broiler and place shrimp on sheet pan 4 inches from broiler and cook for 7 minutes or until they have turned pink. Do not overcook. Remove from oven and let cool slightly. (You can also grill shrimp on an outdoor grill).

Place mixed lettuce and tomatoes in a bowl and toss with ½ cup Sesame Ginger Dressing (see chapter 32). Add shrimp, lightly toss and serve on a platter.

2½ grams carbs; serves 4.

SALAD NICOISE[3]

Phase 1, 2, 3

½ head butter lettuce, broken apart
1 cup black olives, sliced
2 6-oz. cans white albacore tuna
1 cup fresh tomato, chopped
1½ cups celery, chopped
1/2 cup green onions, chopped
2 Tbsp. sunflower seeds
1 16-oz. can great northern beans, rinsed
2 Tbsp. chopped parsley
3 oz. Garlic Herb Dressing (see chapter 32)
2 Tbsp. pine nuts
1 tsp. Herbs de Provence
Sea salt and cracked black pepper to taste

Combine all ingredients nicely on platter. Dress with Garlic Herb Dressing and serve.

17 grams carbs; serves 6.

FIELD GREENS SALAD[4]

Phase 1, 2, 3

4 oz. mixed field greens
1 fresh avocado
1 carrot, shredded
1 tomato, chopped
1 Tbsp. sunflower seeds
½ cup sunflower sprouts

Mix all ingredients in a salad bowl and toss with your choice of Lemon Grape Seed Oil Dressing (see chapter 32) or Garlic Herb Dressing (see chapter 32).

11 grams carbs; serves 4.

SUMMER GREEN SALAD[5]

Phase 1, 2, 3

2 medium fresh tomatoes
4 oz. fresh green beans
1 head endive, quartered and sliced
¾ cup radicchio, shredded
1 Tbsp. raw sunflower seeds
1 Tbsp. olive oil
Sea salt and cracked black pepper to taste
1 Tbsp. fresh herb mix, finely chopped

Chop fresh tomatoes. Steam green beans, and cut into 1-inch pieces. Place in salad serving bowl. Add endive, radicchio, sunflower seeds, olive oil, salt and pepper. Add finely minced fresh parsley, fresh chive, fresh mint or any mixture of your favorite fresh herbs. Toss and serve.

6 grams carbs; serves 4.

INCREDIBLE SUMMER SLAW[6]

Phase 2, 3

2 cups radicchio, shredded
1½ cups endive, sliced
2 cups fresh tomato, chopped
1 lb. fresh cream peas
1 small yellow banana chili pepper
¼ cup fresh cilantro, chopped
½ cup black olives, sliced
⅛ tsp. sea salt
½ tsp. cracked black pepper
2 fresh garlic cloves, minced
¼ tsp. oregano
3 Tbsp. grape seed oil

3 Tbsp. olive oil

2 Tbsp. fresh lemon juice

1 Tbsp. apple cider vinegar

Mix all ingredients in a large bowl. Toss and serve.
13 grams carbs; serves 8.

GARLIC HERB DRESSING[7]

Phase 2, 3

1 cup extra-virgin olive oil

¼ cup Bragg's Apple Cider Vinegar

4 Tbsp. garlic, minced

1 Tbsp. shallots, minced

3 fresh basil leaves, minced

2 tsp. fresh oregano, minced

½ tsp. thyme, minced

½ tsp. fresh parsley, minced

½ tsp. fresh tarragon, minced

½ tsp. fresh mint leaves, minced

Sea salt and cracked black pepper to taste

Mix all ingredients together in pourable container and use as a salad dressing or marinade for poultry or fish. If you prefer a creamier texture, mix ingredients in a blender or small food processor. Keep refrigerated.

This is a versatile dressing. You may substitute dried herbs for fresh, use your own choice of herbs or use lemon instead of apple cider vinegar. Add more herbs for a more intense flavor.

1 gram carbs; makes 1¾ cups.

LEMON GRAPE SEED OIL DRESSING[8]

Phase 2, 3

½ cup grape seed oil

1 cup extra-virgin olive oil

½ cup fresh lemon juice

1 tsp. fresh lemon peel

2 tsp. garlic, chopped

2 Tbsp. shallot, chopped

¼ tsp. white pepper

½ tsp. sea salt

Place all ingredients in a pourable glass container. Shake well and dress with your favorite salad.

1 gram carbs; makes 2½ cups.

CREAMY HERB DRESSING[9]

Phase 2, 3

½ cup pure, cold-pressed safflower oil (from health food store)

1 large tomato, scrubbed and quartered

¼ cup fresh lemon juice

2 large cloves garlic, peeled and crushed

½ tsp. sea salt (optional)

1 Tbsp. each chopped fresh thyme and tarragon

½ tsp. ground paprika

2 Tbsp. 100 percent pure vegetable glycerine

2 Tbsp. sesame seeds

Place all ingredients in a blender, food processor or wide-mouthed jar; mix well. Refrigerate before serving.

18 grams carbs; makes approximately 1 cup.

SAVORY SPANISH DRESSING[10]

Phase 1, 2, 3

1 medium avocado, scrubbed, peeled, pitted and quartered

1 large fresh tomato, scrubbed and quartered

2 large green onions, scrubbed, peeled and cut in half

½ tsp. garlic powder

2 Tbsp. fresh lemon juice

Cayenne pepper to taste

Mix all ingredients in a food processor until creamy; pour over salad.

6 grams carbs; serves 4.

Delicious Homemade Mayonnaise[11]

Phase 2, 3

6 large, pasteurized egg yolks
2 cups pure cold-pressed safflower oil (from health food store)
¼ cup fresh lemon juice
¼ cup water (purified, preferably)
1 tsp. sea salt (optional)
1 tsp. dry mustard

Beat yolks for 2 minutes in a food processor or with an electric mixer. Pour 1 cup of the oil into a measuring cup. Very slowly drizzle a thin stream of oil from the cup into the yolks while beating at high speed until all has been used; mixture should become thick. Drizzle in remaining cup, still beating at high speed. Add lemon juice, water, salt and mustard; mix. Mayonnaise is ready! Spoon mixture into a wide-mouthed quart jar with a tight-fitting lid. Refrigerate until ready to use.

Makes approximately 3 cups.

Sesame Ginger Dressing

Phase 1, 2, 3

¼ cup cold-pressed sesame oil
¼ cup toasted sesame seeds
1½ cups olive oil
⅓ cup Bragg's Liquid Aminos
⅛ cup fresh ginger
⅛ cup fresh garlic, minced
½ Tbsp. red pepper, crushed

Mix all ingredients together and place in salad dressing cruet. Store leftover dressing in refrigerator.

1 gram carbs; makes 2½ cups.

Chapter 33

ENTICING ENTRÉES

CHICKEN CUTLETS ITALIANO[1]
Phase 1, 2, 3

¼ cup extra-virgin olive oil
2 organic eggs
⅓ cup brown rice flour
4 chicken cutlets (breast halves, skinned and boned)
1 cup scrubbed zucchini, sliced in ⅛-inch rounds
1 tsp. garlic powder, more or less, to taste
1 Tbsp. chopped fresh oregano
1 8-oz. can unsweetened tomato sauce (without citric acid)

Heat oil in a large nonstick skillet. Beat eggs in a small bowl. Spoon flour into a pie dish. Dip chicken breasts first into egg, next into flour and then place in skillet; add zucchini. Sprinkle half of the seasonings over top; brown over medium-high heat. Turn; reduce heat. Spoon tomato sauce over cutlets and zucchini. Sprinkle remaining half of the seasonings over sauce. Simmer, covered, 10–15 minutes, or until fork-tender.

16 grams carbs; serves 4.

GREEK-STYLE BREAST OF CHICKEN[2]
Phase 1, 2, 3

½ cup extra-virgin olive oil
Juice of 1 medium lemon, scrubbed before slicing
Chopped fresh oregano to taste
Garlic powder to taste
2–4 chicken breast halves, skinned, with bones

Place a small bowl and foil-lined broiling pan next to each other. Place oil, lemon juice and seasonings in bowl; mix. Dip both sides of chicken into the lemon-olive oil mixture and then place in broiling pan, reserving leftover sauce for basting. Broil one side until browned (about 5 minutes), basting often. Turn; broil other side, basting frequently until chicken is fork-tender.

2–3 grams carbs; serves 2–4.

CAJUN CHICKEN BREAST[3]

Phase 1, 2, 3

4 4-oz. boneless, skinless chicken breasts
1 Tbsp. olive oil
2 Tbsp. Cajun spice mix

Coat chicken breasts with olive oil and spice mix. Place in oven and broil for 20 minutes, turning after 10 minutes. Instead of broiling, you can also grill these chicken breasts using your favorite method.

½ grams carbs; serves 4.

GARLIC CHICKEN AND PASTA[4]

Phase 1, 2, 3

2–3 Tbsp. extra-virgin olive oil (enough for sautéing)
1 cup chicken broth
1–2 cloves garlic, minced (to taste)
1–2 Tbsp. minced onion or shallot (to taste)
Salt and pepper (to taste)
½ lemon
2 skinless chicken breasts, cut up
½ lb. cooked spelt pasta

Melt butter and olive oil in pan and sauté onion/shallot and garlic over low to medium heat until well caramelized. Add chicken and brown on all sides. Add chicken broth, salt and pepper. Lower heat and simmer until liquid is reduced by half. Squeeze ½ lemon over chicken and toss in cooked spelt pasta.

Note: For variation, add other vegetables such as squash, zucchini, broccoli, tomatoes, etc.

42 grams carbs; serves 4.

TURKEY AND WILD RICE CASSEROLE[5]

Phase 1, 2, 3

1 cup raw wild rice
¼ cup extra-virgin olive oil
1 medium yellow onion, scrubbed, peeled and chopped
1 medium green bell pepper, scrubbed and diced
2 stalks celery, scrubbed and thinly sliced
¾ pound fresh natural turkey breast, cubed
8 oz. canned water chestnuts, drained and sliced
1 17½-oz. can unsweetened chicken broth
1 Tbsp. potato or brown rice flour
1 tsp. garlic powder
1 tsp. chopped fresh sage

Preheat oven to 350 degrees. Rinse wild rice twice in colander under cold running water. Heat oil in an 8-inch nonstick skillet. Add onion, pepper, celery and turkey; sauté until browned. Add water chestnuts, rice and broth; mix. Add flour and seasonings; mix until well blended. Pour mixture into a 3-quart casserole dish. Cover; bake 45 minutes.

31 grams carbs; serves 6.

SHRIMP AND CHICKEN JAMBALAYA[6]

Phase 1, 2, 3

2 Tbsp. extra-virgin olive oil
4 cloves garlic, chopped
⅓ cup green onion, chopped
⅓ cup red onion, diced
⅓ cup each of yellow, red and green bell pepper, diced
¼ cup celery, diced
¼ cup fresh parsley
¼ tsp. thyme

2 cups short-grain brown rice
4¾ cups chicken stock
1¾ Tbsp. Cajun spice (read label)
3 Tbsp. butter
1¼ lb. chicken breast, cubed
1¼ lb. shrimp, peeled and deveined
Sea salt and pepper to taste

Sauté chicken and shrimp in butter and set aside in a bowl. Add salt and pepper to taste. In same pan, heat olive oil; add garlic and vegetables and sauté until translucent. Add rice and sauté for 5 minutes.

Add chicken stock and spice; cook until rice is tender. Add chicken and shrimp and toss, adding water if necessary. Serve in large bowls.

40 grams carbs; serves 6.

ORANGE ROUGHY WITH SPECIAL BUTTER SAUCE AND ALMONDS[7]

Phase 1, 2, 3

½ cup clarified or organic butter
1 tsp. each chopped fresh basil and oregano
Garlic powder to taste
4 orange roughy fillets (6–8 ounces each)
½ cup sliced or ground fresh almonds
1 medium lemon, scrubbed and cut into wedges, for garnish
Fresh parsley sprigs for garnish

Preheat oven to 350 degrees. Melt butter in a small skillet; add seasonings, mix and immediately remove from heat. Dip both sides of fish into butter sauce; place in a baking dish and pour any remaining sauce over tops of fillets. Sprinkle almonds over top. Bake 20 minutes. Test for doneness with a fork. Garnish with lemon and parsley.

7 grams carbs; serves 4.

FLORENTINE-STUFFED SOLE[8]

Phase 1, 2, 3

1 10-oz. package frozen spinach, chopped
½ cup clarified or organic butter or extra-virgin olive oil
1 tsp. garlic powder
1 tsp. each chopped fresh basil and oregano
½ tsp. ground nutmeg
4 sole fillets (6–8 ounces each)
½ cup sliced or ground fresh raw almonds
1 medium lemon, scrubbed and sliced, for garnish
Fresh parsley sprigs, for garnish

Preheat oven to 350 degrees. Thaw spinach in a microwave or colander; drain and squeeze out any liquid. Heat butter or oil in a large nonstick skillet; add spinach and seasonings. Mix well and remove from heat. Place spinach on the center of each fillet, reserving butter sauce in skillet. Roll fillets; secure with toothpicks. Place fillets into a greased 8-inch baking dish. Mix almonds into butter sauce; sprinkle over fillet tops. Bake 20 minutes; fillets are done when they flake at the touch of a fork. Garnish with lemons and parsley.

6 grams carbs; serves 4.

MEAT MARINADE[9]

Phase 2, 3

1 large clove garlic
2 Tbsp. lemon juice
1 Tbsp. raw unpasteurized apple cider vinegar
1½ tsp. steak spice
½ tsp. celery salt
2 Tbsp. extra-virgin olive oil
½ tsp. salt

Mix all ingredients together and coat meat before cooking. This can be used to marinate chicken breasts or on beef in a Crock-Pot. This recipe can easily be doubled.

2½ grams carbs.

SPECIAL SPAGHETTI AND SAUCE[10]

Phase 1, 2, 3

1 15-oz. can unsweetened tomato sauce (without citric acid)
1 6-oz. can tomato paste (without citric acid)
2 Tbsp. coarsely chopped fresh parsley
2 Tbsp. extra-virgin olive oil
1 Tbsp. each coarsely chopped fresh basil and oregano
1 7-oz. package cooked and drained soba, spelt or rice noodles

Place sauce ingredients in a large kettle; heat. Bring to a boil; cover and simmer 1 hour. Serve over noodles.

51 grams carbs; serves 4.

QUICK MARINARA SAUCE[11]

Phase 1, 2, 3

2 tsp. extra-virgin olive oil
1 28-oz. can crushed tomatoes (without citric acid)
6 cloves garlic, sliced
4 fresh basil leaves
1 tsp. cracked black pepper
Sea salt to taste

Place olive oil in a saucepan and heat slightly. Add sliced garlic and sauté. Do not brown. Remove pan from heat and pour in crushed tomatoes. Place over heat again and simmer for 5 minutes. Add chopped basil leaves. Add pepper and salt to taste.

16 grams carbs; makes 3½ cups.

HAMBURGERS[12]

Phase 1, 2, 3

1¼ lb. lean free-range ground sirloin
1 tsp. cracked black pepper
1 tsp. Wesbrae Un-Ketchup
4 millet hamburger buns, cut in half, and grilled, broiled or toasted

Mix ingredients except buns together and divide into four 5-oz. patties. Heat broiler. Broil burgers, 4 inches from broiler, until desired doneness is reached. Approximate times: 6 minutes, rare; 8 minutes, medium rare; 10 minutes, well done. Turn burgers halfway through the cooking process.

Place burgers on buns and top with choice of sliced tomato, onion, ketchup (see chapter 37), lettuce, pico de gallo (see chapter 37), guacamole, pepper rings, green grilled onions or salsa. (Phase 2, add Vegenaise.)

Burgers may also be grilled or pan-fried.

40 grams carbs; serves 4.

TEXAS BEEF AND ROASTED CHILI[13]

Phase 1, 2, 3

2 Tbsp. extra-virgin olive oil

3 large onions, chopped

2 lb. extra-lean free range ground beef

4 Tbsp. chili powder

3 Tbsp. cumin powder

1 Tbsp. granulated garlic

1 Tbsp. cayenne pepper

1 Tbsp. cracked black pepper

1 28-oz. can crushed tomatoes (without citric acid)

3 lb. green chili peppers, roasted

In a large Crock-Pot, heat olive oil and sauté onions until translucent. Add ground beef and all spices. Cook until beef is browned. Add tomatoes and simmer for 1 hour.

In the meantime, roast chili peppers. Chop peppers, then stir into beef mixture. Heat and serve.

34 grams carbs; serves 10.

SHEPHERD'S PIE[14]

Phase 1, 2, 3

2½ lb. lean free-range ground beef
1 Tbsp. extra-virgin olive oil
4 garlic cloves, chopped
1 cup onions, chopped
1 cup red bell pepper, chopped
1 tsp. cracked black pepper
½ tsp. garlic powder
¼ tsp. rosemary
¼ tsp. sage
¼ tsp. tarragon
2 cups petite green peas (frozen), heated
1 large head cauliflower, trimmed into florets
Pinch sea salt
¼ tsp. white pepper

In a sauté pan, brown ground beef; drain and set aside.

In the same pan, add olive oil, garlic, onions and peppers; sauté until soft. Add spices and ground beef; let simmer on low heat for about 10 minutes, then remove from heat.

Steam trimmed cauliflower until tender; drain well and pat dry. Place cauliflower in a food processor and puree until it reaches the consistency of mashed potatoes.

Season with sea salt and white pepper.

10 grams carbs; serves 8.

BRAISED BEEF[15]

Phase 1, 2, 3

2½ lb. boneless free-range chuck roast
2 cups beef broth
1½ Tbsp. garlic, minced (about 6 cloves)
2 bay leafs
1 tsp. oregano
3 medium onions, diced
2 large celery stalks, diced

2 medium red bell peppers
1 tsp. rosemary, finely chopped
1 28-oz. can whole tomatoes, chopped in food processor
1½ tsp. cracked black pepper
¼ tsp. sea salt
2 Tbsp. extra-virgin olive oil
2 Tbsp. arrowroot (thickener)

Preheat over to 425 degrees.

Heat olive oil in roasting pan, brown roast, add vegetables, and sauté lightly about 10 minutes. Add other ingredients except arrowroot. Cover and place in oven. Cook until meat is fork tender.

Remove meat and skim fat; reduce sauce by ¼ on stovetop and thicken with arrowroot. Return meat to sauce.

For variety, try lamb, veal or pork shanks with the same preparation. (This is a great recipe for the Crock-Pot.)

19 grams carbs; serves 6.

GRILLED CHICKEN FAJITAS[16]

Phase 1, 2, 3

2 lb. boneless, skinless chicken breasts and thighs
2 Tbsp. extra-virgin olive oil
1 tsp. granulated garlic
½ tsp. sea salt
1 tsp. cracked black pepper
1 tsp. cumin powder

Cut chicken into strips. Place in bowl and add all ingredients. Marinate for 30 minutes. Heat broiler, and place chicken 4 inches from broiler. Cook for 15 minutes, turning as necessary.

Serve with warmed spelt tortillas, pico de gallo (see chapter 37), guacamole and sautéed peppers and onions.

1 gram carbs; serves 4.

Chapter 34

VIRTUOUS VEGETABLES

SPANISH BROWN RICE[1]

Phase 1, 2, 3

1 cup water (purified, preferably)
½ cup raw brown rice
¼ tsp. sea salt (optional)
2 Tbsp. extra-virgin olive oil
1 medium yellow onion, scrubbed, peeled and chopped
1 medium green bell pepper, scrubbed and chopped
½ cup chopped fresh parsley
2 large fresh tomatoes, scrubbed, peeled, cored and coarsely chopped
Cayenne pepper to taste

Bring water to a boil in a 1-quart saucepan. Add rice and salt. Reduce heat, cover and simmer 40 minutes, or until all liquid is absorbed. Heat oil in a large nonstick skillet. Add rice and rest of ingredients. Sauté over medium-high heat, stirring frequently until vegetables are tender.

26 grams carbs; serves 4.

CAJUN RICE[2]

Phase 1, 2, 3

2 cups short-grain brown rice
2 Tbsp. extra-virgin olive oil
2 Tbsp. garlic, chopped
¼ cup celery, chopped
⅓ cup red bell peppers
⅓ cup yellow bell peppers

½ cup green bell peppers
¼ tsp. fresh thyme
½ tsp. crushed red pepper
1¾ Tbsp. Cajun seasoning mix
5 cups chicken broth
¼ cup parsley, chopped

Heat olive oil in a saucepan and add garlic, celery and peppers. Sauté until slightly cooked and soft. Add rice and thyme and sauté until rice is shiny, about 4 minutes. Add crushed red pepper and Cajun seasoning mix and stir. Add chicken broth and bring to a boil. Reduce heat and simmer covered for 45 minutes or until rice is cooked. Remove from heat and stir in parsley.

Note: Serve with a main meal or add to a soup or stew.

35 grams carbs; serves 10.

WILD RICE AND ALMONDS[3]

Phase 1, 2, 3

1 cup raw wild rice
3 cups water (purified, preferably)
1 tsp. sea salt (optional)
2 Tbsp. extra-virgin olive oil
1 large clove garlic, scrubbed, peeled and minced
2 stalks celery, without leaves, scrubbed and coarsely chopped
1 medium yellow onion, scrubbed, peeled and coarsely chopped
½ cup chopped fresh parsley
½ cup slivered or ground fresh almonds

Boil wild rice with 2 cups water for 1 minute; drain. Repeat process. Then place rice, 3 cups water and salt in a 3-quart saucepan. Cover and simmer 35 minutes or until kernels puff open; drain. Pour oil into a large skillet, sauté garlic, celery, onion and parsley until tender. Add almonds and cooked rice; mix well. Simmer, covered, 15 minutes, or place rice mixture into a greased mold and bake in a preheated 350-degree oven for 20–30 minutes. Serve hot with entrée.

25 grams carbs; serves 4.

BROCCOLI ITALIAN STYLE[4]

Phase 1, 2, 3

1 head broccoli
2 Tbsp. extra-virgin olive oil
¼ tsp. granulated garlic
⅛ tsp. sea salt
¼ tsp. cracked black pepper
¼ tsp. sesame seeds

Separate broccoli florets and cut stems to about 1½ inches or more. Steam until cooked to desired tenderness. Remove from steamer and arrange on serving platter. While still hot, drizzle olive oil over florets, then sprinkle garlic, salt, black pepper and sesame seeds over florets. Serve at room temperature.

8 grams carbs; serves 4.

GREEN BEANS PALERMO[5]

Phase 1, 2, 3

1 lb. fresh green beans
1½ tsp. extra virgin olive oil
2 garlic cloves, chopped
Sea salt and cracked black pepper to taste

Cut ends off green beans and wash thoroughly. Steam beans until desired tenderness is reached, approximately 10 minutes. Heat olive oil in sauté pan and cook garlic. Do not brown. Add green beans and toss in pan until coated. Remove from heat and place on serving dish. Add salt and pepper to taste. This dish can be served hot, cold or at room temperature.

4 grams carbs; serves 8.

HACIENDA PINTO BEANS[6]

Phase 1, 2, 3

2 cups dry beans* (or 2 15-oz. cans)
6 cups water (reduce 3 cups if using canned beans)
2 cups onion, chopped
4 cloves fresh garlic, chopped
2 cups fresh tomatoes, chopped
½ cup fresh cilantro, chopped
2 jalapenos, chopped
½ tsp. crushed red pepper
1 Tbsp. cumin
1 Tbsp. oregano

* Soak beans according to package directions.

In a stockpot, heat olive oil. Add onion and garlic, and sauté lightly. Add water, beans and rest of ingredients. Simmer for 2 hours. (If using canned beans, simmer for about 1 hour.)

34 grams carbs; serves 10.

BRAISED CABBAGE AND PEAS[7]

Phase 1, 2, 3

1 head green cabbage (about 6 cups, sliced)
1–2 Tbsp. extra-virgin olive oil
2 Tbsp. chopped garlic
1 cup chicken broth
½ cup chopped parsley
1 cup frozen green peas
½ tsp. black pepper

Heat extra-virgin olive oil in sauté pan and add chopped garlic. Sauté garlic slightly and add cabbage. Cover and steam for 5 minutes. Add chicken broth. Reduce heat to simmer and braise for about 10 minutes. Stir in parsley and frozen peas; cover and cook for an additional 5 minutes or until the cabbage is tender. Season with pepper.

8½ grams carbs; serves 6.

ASPARAGUS SAUTÉ[8]

Phase 1, 2, 3

1 lb. fresh, thin asparagus, scrubbed and cut on the diagonal into 2-inch pieces
Water (purified, preferably)
2 Tbsp. extra-virgin olive oil
Grated, scrubbed fresh ginger root to taste
2 large cloves garlic, scrubbed, peeled and minced
½ tsp. sea salt (optional)
2 Tbsp. sesame seeds

Place asparagus in a large pot; cover with water. Bring to a boil, reduce heat, and cook 5 minutes. Heat oil in a large skillet. Add ginger, garlic, salt, sesame seeds and asparagus. Sauté, stirring and turning frequently, until tender.
3 grams carbs; serves 4.

SAVORY LIMA BEANS[9]

Phase 1, 2, 3

1 lb. dried lima beans, washed thoroughly, soaked overnight and drained
Water (purified, preferably)
2 Tbsp. extra-virgin olive oil
1 medium yellow onion, scrubbed, peeled and coarsely chopped
1 large clove garlic, scrubbed, peeled and minced
2 Tbsp. garbanzo flour
Cayenne pepper to taste
1 tsp. sea salt (optional)
1 8-oz. can unsweetened tomato sauce (without citric acid)
1 6-oz. can tomato paste (without citric acid)
1 Tbsp. 100 percent pure vegetable glycerine

Preheat oven to 350 degrees. Place beans in a large kettle; cover with water. Bring to a boil; lower heat and simmer 2 minutes; drain. Repeat process twice more. Add water to cover beans; simmer covered, 30 minutes. Sauté onion and garlic in oil until tender. Place garlic, onion, beans with liquid and rest of ingredients in an 8-inch casserole dish; mix. Bake 45 minutes or until tender.
23½ grams carbs; serves 6.

Chapter 35

DELICIOUS DESSERTS

Tapioca Pudding[1]

Phrase 2, 3

3 Tbsp. Minute Tapioca (gluten-free)
⅛ tsp. Stevia
½ tsp. salt
2 cups unsweetened soy, almond or rice milk
1 organic egg, divided
1 tsp. vanilla

Beat egg white until light and fluffy. In a saucepan, over medium heat, combine milk, Stevia and vanilla. Heat until hot, then stir some of the soy milk into the egg yolk. Return to saucepan and add tapioca. Cook about 10 minutes, stirring constantly so it won't scorch. When thickened, fold in the egg white. Pour into four serving bowls.

8 grams carbs; serves 4.

Pumpkin and Pecan Loaf[2]

Phase 2, 3

2 large organic eggs, beaten
⅓ cup clarified or organic butter
¼ cup 100 percent pure vegetable glycerine
2 cups canned unsweetened pumpkin
1¼ cups brown rice flour
½ tsp. sea salt (optional)
2 tsp. baking powder
½ tsp. ground cloves

½ tsp. each ground cinnamon, ginger and nutmeg
½ cup chopped or ground fresh pecans

Preheat oven to 350 degrees. Mix all ingredients except nuts in a large bowl until well blended. Mix in pecans. Pour batter into a 5- x 9-inch loaf pan well oiled with extra-virgin olive oil and lightly floured. Bake 50–60 minutes. Test for doneness with a toothpick. Cool before slicing.
23 grams carbs; makes 12 slices.

MIXED BERRY COMPOTE[3]

Phase 2, 3

1 cup unsweetened blueberries, frozen
1 cup unsweetened strawberries, frozen
1 cup unsweetened blackberries, frozen
1 cup water
¹⁄₁₆ tsp. pure Stevia powder
2 tsp. arrowroot powder

Place berries and ¾ cup water in a small saucepan; cook about 15 minutes. Add Stevia, and taste for sweetness. Add more for desired sweetness, ¹⁄₁₆ tsp. at a time. Mix ¼ cup water with arrowroot powder and add to mixture; simmer until thickened. Remove from heat. Serve with pancakes or waffles.
10 grams carbs; makes 3 cups.

DARK CHOCOLATE ALMOND TRUFFLES[4]

Phase 2, 3

¾ cup almond butter
½ cup crushed almonds or pecans
3 Pure De-lite Dark Chocolate bars
¼ cup dried flaked unsweetened coconut

Line a sheet pan (or pan that can go in the freezer) with parchment paper. Freeze almond butter for 2 hours. With tip of teaspoon or melon ball tool approximately ½ teaspoon size, make small almond butter ball. Cover each ball completely with crushed almonds and place on sheet pan, leaving about 1½ inches between balls. Place back in freezer while preparing the chocolate.

Break up chocolate into 1-inch pieces. Place into a microwave-safe non-plastic container. Microwave chocolate in 40-second intervals, stirring each time, until chocolate is melted and ribbons off spoon. Do not overheat.

Take almond balls from freezer. With a teaspoon, drizzle chocolate over almond ball until the ball is completely and smoothly covered. Sprinkle with coconut, then place back in freezer until ready to serve.

5 grams carbs; makes 12 truffles, ½ oz. each.

APPLE CINNAMON BREAD PUDDING[5]

Phase 2, 3

8 oz. green apples, sliced

1 large egg

1½ cups soy or coconut or rice milk

14 slices millet bread, cubed

¼ cup dark agave nectar

½ tsp. cinnamon

¼ tsp. allspice

¼ tsp. ginger

½ tsp. butter to coat baking pan

Mix egg, milk and spices until incorporated. Add cubed bread and soak until mixture is absorbed. Add more milk if too dry. Fold in apples. Place in buttered glass baking dish. Bake at 350 degrees for 25 minutes until top is browned.

40 grams carbs; serves 6.

LEMON AND PECAN COOKIES[6]

Phase 2, 3

½ cup clarified or organic butter

3 Tbsp. 100 percent pure vegetable glycerine

1 large organic egg

1½ cups + 4½ tsp. brown rice flour

½ tsp. baking soda

1¼ cup fresh lemon juice

2 Tbsp. lemon flavoring
½ cup chopped or ground pecans

Preheat oven to 375 degrees. Mix butter and glycerine in a large bowl. Add egg, flour and baking soda; mix well. Fold in lemon juice, flavoring and pecans. Drop rounded teaspoonfuls of dough onto a nonstick cookie sheet. Bake 8–10 minutes. Cool 5 minutes before removing from cookie sheet. 12 grams carbs; makes 2 dozen cookies.

NUT BUTTER COOKIES[7]

Phase 2, 3

¼ cup clarified or organic butter, melted
½ cup Delicious and Easy Nut Butter (see chapter 37)
2 Tbsp. 100 percent pure vegetable glycerine
⅓ cup unsweetened soy milk
1 large organic egg
1 tsp. vanilla flavoring
1¼ cups sifted brown rice flour
1 tsp. baking powder
¼ tsp. sea salt (optional)
2 dozen fresh pecans or walnuts, cut into halves or ground

Preheat oven to 350 degrees. Combine butters, glycerine, milk, egg and flavoring in a large bowl. Place dry ingredients in another large bowl; mix together. Add dry mixture to milk mixture; blend well. Place teaspoonfuls of dough on a nonstick cookie sheet; flatten cookies with back of spoon; press nut halves into tops. Bake 8–10 minutes. Let cookies cool for 5 minutes before removing them from cookie sheet. Cookies will harden as they cool.
5 grams carbs; makes 4 dozen cookies.

PUMPKIN COOKIES[8]

Phase 2, 3

1 cup canned unsweetened pumpkin
½ cup clarified or organic butter
¼ cup 100 percent pure vegetable glycerine
1 Tbsp. orange flavoring
1½ cups brown rice flour
1 tsp. baking soda
1 tsp. ground cinnamon
¼ tsp. sea salt (optional)
½ cup chopped or ground fresh walnuts

Preheat oven to 375 degrees. Mix pumpkin, butter, glycerine and orange flavoring in a large bowl. Add flour, baking soda and seasonings; mix. Fold in nuts. Place teaspoonfuls on a nonstick cookie sheet. Bake 8–10 minutes or until lightly browned. Let cookies stand for 5 minutes before removing them from cookie sheet. They will harden as they cool.

8 grams carbs; makes 3 dozen cookies.

Chapter 36

SCRUMPTIOUS SOUPS, SNACKS AND APPETIZERS

SAVORY BLACK BEAN SOUP[1]

Phase 1, 2, 3

1 cup raw black beans, washed thoroughly, soaked overnight and drained
1 quart water (purified, preferably)
1 Tbsp. coarsely chopped fresh parsley
¾ tsp. ground turmeric
⅛ tsp. ground cumin
1 tsp. each chopped fresh marjoram and thyme
2 Tbsp. extra-virgin olive oil
2 large cloves garlic, scrubbed, peeled and minced
1 medium yellow onion, scrubbed, peeled and finely chopped
2 stalks celery, without leaves, scrubbed and finely chopped
1 6-oz. can tomato paste (without citric acid)
Sea salt to taste (optional)

Place beans in a large kettle; cover with water. Bring to a boil; cook 2 minutes; drain. Repeat boiling process twice more. Then place 1 quart water, beans, spices and herbs in kettle; bring to a boil. Simmer uncovered, 30 minutes. Spoon beans and their liquid into blender; blend until creamy. Place mixture in kettle; bring to a boil; simmer, uncovered. Heat oil in a small skillet. Sauté garlic and onion until tender; add with tomato paste to beans. Mix; cook uncovered 10 minutes and serve.

29 grams carbs; serves 6.

LENTIL SOUP AND MEATBALLS[2]

Phase 1, 2, 3

3 Tbsp. olive oil
3 celery stalks, chopped
1 large onion, chopped
3 cloves garlic, chopped
8 cups water
2 cups lentils (washed and rinsed thoroughly)
1 tsp. thyme
1 tsp. sea salt
1 tsp. cracked black pepper
1 cup baby spinach

Heat olive oil in stockpot. Add celery, onion and garlic; sauté until tender. Add water, lentils and spices. Simmer until the lentils are tender—approximately 1 hour. Add spinach and meatballs; simmer for 15 minutes.

Meatballs:

½ lb. ground sirloin, pork or veal
1 tsp. cracked black pepper
½ tsp. sea salt
¼ tsp. crushed red pepper

Mix all ingredients thoroughly in a bowl. Form into small ½-inch meatballs and drop into simmer soup.

23 grams carbs; serves 10.

MINESTRONE[3]

Phase 1, 2, 3

2 Tbsp. olive oil
4 cloves garlic, chopped
1 medium onion, chopped
2 celery stalks with leaves, chopped
2 cups green cabbage
1 28-oz. can whole tomatoes, chopped in food processor
4 cups water (more or less for desired heartiness of soup)

2 cups fresh baby spinach

¼ cup fresh basil, chopped

¼ cup fresh parsley, chopped

1 tsp. rosemary

¼ tsp. oregano

1 can white beans, rinsed

Sea salt and cracked black pepper to taste

Heat olive oil in stockpot. Add garlic, onion, celery and cabbage; sauté until vegetables are tender. Add tomatoes, water and spices; simmer for 30–45 minutes. Add spinach and white beans. Stir and simmer for 5 minutes until spinach is wilted and soup is thoroughly heated.

16 grams carbohydrates per serving; serves 12.

CHICKEN AND RICE SOUP[4]

Phase 1, 2, 3

1 chicken, skinned and cut up

2 quarts water or broth

4 cloves garlic, sliced (optional, to taste)

2 cups each celery, carrots, onions, peas (sliced)

½ cup cooked brown rice

½ cup parsley, chopped

Herbs and seasoning to taste

Simmer chicken in water or stock for 40 minutes. Add vegetables and rice; simmer for 20 additional minutes. Serve broth and vegetables with chicken meat. Top with scissor-snipped fresh parsley. Add herbs according to taste.

Variation: ¼ cup raw rice may be added to water and simmered with chicken.

12 grams carbs; serves 10.

GAZPACHO SOUP[5]

Phase 1, 2, 3

3 cups tomato juice (read labels)
6 cups V-8 juice (low sodium, read label)
1 Tbsp. cracked black pepper
1 tsp. sea salt
¼ tsp. cayenne pepper
¼ cup olive oil
2 cups beef stock (can use vegetable or chicken stock)
1 Tbsp. ground cumin
1 tsp. Bragg's Amino Acid
2 tsp. chili powder
2 tsp. minced garlic
2 Tbsp. fresh cilantro, chopped (for garnish)
1 cucumber, chopped (for garnish)

Combine all ingredients in food processor and pulse until combined. Place in large bowl and chill for 2 hours. Serve in chilled bowls.

9 grams carbs; serves 12.

GUACAMOLE[6]

Phase 1, 2, 3

16 oz. avocados or 1 pkg. Hass Avocado Halves
8-oz. pkg. Avo Green Salsa
2 Tbsp. fresh cilantro, chopped
1 small fresh tomato, chopped
½ small red onion, chopped
Sea salt

Crush avocados and mix in all ingredients or pulse in food processor. Add sea salt to taste.

5 grams carbs; makes 2½ cups.

BLACK BEAN DIP[7]

Phase 1, 2, 3

1 15-oz. can black beans (drained and rinsed)
2 medium fresh tomatoes, chopped
½ cup cilantro, chopped
⅓ cup white onion, chopped
2 small serrano peppers, minced
1 Tbsp. lime juice

Place all ingredients in food processor and process until desired consistency is reached.

11 grams carbs; serves 6.

HUMMUS[8]

Phase 1, 2, 3

1 15-oz. chickpeas (garbanzo beans), drained
2 Tbsp. olive oil
1 Tbsp. sesame oil
¼ tsp. cracked black pepper
1 tsp. fresh garlic
2 Tbsp. water

Mix all ingredients in a small food processor until smooth. Serve with Belgian endive or Edward & Sons Brown Rice Crackers.

11 grams carbs; serves 8.

GARLIC BREAD[9]

Phase 2, 3

16 thinly sliced ¼-inch "O" spelt sourdough bread
½ tsp. extra-virgin olive oil
¼ tsp. granulated garlic
¼ tsp. cracked black pepper
1¼ tsp. oregano
¼ tsp. red pepper, crushed

Place bread on sheet pan, spray with olive oil, and sprinkle each slice with spice mixture. Place about 4 inches from broiler and broil for about 3–4 minutes until browned.

22 grams carbs; serves 8.

QUINOA TABOULI[10]

Phase 1, 2, 3

1½ cup quinoa
2 medium cucumbers, skinned, seeded and chopped
½ cup fresh parsley, chopped
2 Tbsp. fresh lemon juice
1 tsp. fresh garlic, chopped
1 Tbsp. olive oil
Sea salt and pepper

Cook quinoa according to package directions. Let cool. Add cucumbers, parsley, lemon juice, garlic, olive oil, salt and pepper. Mix all ingredients thoroughly and chill.

47 grams carbs; serves 4.

Chapter 37

AND THAT'S NOT ALL!

KETCHUP[1]

Phase 1, 2, 3

1 cup Westbrae Unsweetened Un-Ketchup
1/16 tsp. pure Stevia powder

Mix to combine ingredients. Use as you would regular ketchup.
0 grams carbs; serves 4.

ALMOND MILK[2]

Phase 2, 3

1 cup fresh raw almonds
2 cups boiling water (purified, preferably)
1 quart cold water (purified, preferably)
1 Tbsp. pure, cold-pressed safflower oil from health food store
2 Tbsp. 100 percent pure vegetable glycerine
1/4 tsp. sea salt (optional)

Blanch almonds by pouring boiling water over nuts; soak a few minutes
or until skins slide off easily; drain. Place skinless almonds, cold water, oil,
glycerine and salt in a food processor or blender. Process to a very smooth
liquid. If necessary, strain with cheesecloth or a fine strainer; refrigerate. Use
in recipes as you would pasteurized or soy milk.
4 grams carbs; makes approximately 1 quart.

MOCK SOUR CREAM[3]

Phase 2, 3

1 cup plain low-fat, lactose-free yogurt
1 tsp. 100 percent pure vegetable glycerine

Mix yogurt and glycerine in a small bowl. Chill at least 30 minutes before serving.
12 grams carbs; makes approximately 1 cup.

PICO DE GALLO[4]

Phase 1, 2, 3

2½ cups fresh tomatoes, diced
1 cup onion, diced
½ cup cilantro, chopped
½ cup serrano peppers, minced
Pinch sea salt
Squeeze of lemon juice

Mix all ingredients in a bowl. Chill and serve as a condiment with beans and fajitas.
5 grams carbs; serves 4–6.

BÉARNAISE II SAUCE[5]

Phase 2, 3

1½ Tbsp. Bragg's Apple Cider Vinegar
1 shallot, finely minced
½ tsp. cracked black pepper
1½ Tbsp. tarragon
2 Tbsp. lemon juice
½ cup clarified butter
3 organic egg yolks
1½ Tbsp. water
½ tsp. sea salt

In a small saucepan over medium heat, combine apple cider vinegar, shallot, pepper, tarragon, lemon juice and ½ Tbsp. water. Simmer until reduced by ⅓. Remove from heat.

In the upper section of a double boiler, off heat, whisk egg yolks and cold water until frothy. Place the pan over the barely simmer water of the bottom section and continue whisking egg yolks for 3–4 minutes until eggs are thickened. Do not let eggs get too hot or they will scramble.

When eggs are thickened, remove pan from heat and slowly whisk in warm clarified butter. Whisk in the reduced tarragon liquid until sauce is smooth and incorporated. Keep covered until ready to serve.

1 gram carbs; makes 1 cup.

COCKTAIL SAUCE[6]

Phase 1, 2, 3

1 cup Westbrae Unsweetened Un-Ketchup
¹⁄₁₆ tsp. white Stevia powder
½ tsp. Bragg's Amino Acids
1 Tbsp. organic horseradish

Mix all ingredients together in a bowl. Garnish with fresh herbs. Use more or less horseradish to your taste.

10 grams carbs; serves 6.

CAJUN NUT MIX[7]

Phase 1, 2, 3

1 cup raw hulled sunflower seeds
1 cup soy nuts
1 cup pecan halves
1 cup pumpkin seeds
1 cup almonds
1 Tbsp. Cajun seasoning mix (be sure to check the label for "illegal" additives)
Extra-virgin olive oil
Sea salt

Preheat oven to 350 degrees. Lightly spray olive oil onto a sheet pan. Place nuts and seeds on pan, and spray them lightly with olive oil. Sprinkle seasoning and salt to lightly coat mixture. Roast mixture until lightly browned, approximately 15 minutes. Turn halfway through the cooking process. Remove from oven and reseason. Let cool completely. Place in glass bowl or jar. Store in airtight container and refrigerate.

40 grams carbs; 10-plus servings.

SALT-FREE CHILI POWDER[8]

Phase 1, 2, 3

2 Tbsp. paprika
2 tsp. oregano
1¼ tsp. ground cumin
1¼ tsp. garlic powder
¾ tsp. cayenne pepper
¾ tsp. onion powder

Combine all ingredients; mix thoroughly. Store in airtight container.
1 gram carbs per teaspoon; makes ¼ cup.

CREOLE SEASONING[9]

Phase 1, 2, 3

8 tsp. salt
2 Tbsp. pepper
2 Tbsp. garlic powder
8 tsp. paprika
8 tsp. cayenne pepper
4½ tsp. onion powder
1 Tbsp. thyme
2 Tbsp. grated lemon rind

In a screw-top jar, combine all ingredients. Shake thoroughly to mix. Keep in a dry place.

¾ grams carbs; makes ¾ cup.

DELICIOUS AND EASY NUT BUTTER[10]

Phase 1, 2, 3

½ cup fresh raw pecans, walnuts or almonds

1 tablespoon cold-pressed safflower oil (from health food store)

Combine nuts and oil in a food processor or blender; mix until creamy. Spread on rice cakes or rice crackers or use in recipes.

1¾ grams carbs per teaspoon

APPENDIX A
THE BIBLE CURE'S SIMPLE
RULES FOR WEIGHT LOSS
(From *The New Bible Cure for Weight Loss*)

THE FOLLOWING ARE simple dieting rules that I always recommend to my patients who need to lose weight:

1. Graze throughout the day. (Eat lots of salads and veggies often throughout the day, and eat beans, peas, or lentils once or twice a day, up to four cups daily.)

2. Eat a large breakfast. As the saying goes, eat breakfast like a king, lunch like a prince, and dinner like a pauper. Eat smaller midmorning and midafternoon snacks.

3. Avoid all simple-sugar foods, i.e., candies, cookies, cakes, pies, and doughnuts. If you must have sugar, use either stevia, xylitol, Sweet Balance, Just Like Sugar (found in health food stores), or small amounts of coconut sugar or tagatose.

4. Drink two quarts of filtered or bottled water a day. That includes 16 ounces thirty minutes before each meal, or one to two 8-ounce glasses two and a half hours after each meal. Also, drink 8 to 16 ounces of water upon awakening.

5. Avoid alcohol and all fried foods.

6. For meals, choose a lean protein, a low-glycemic carb, and a healthy fat (but do your best to go "carb free" and low fat after 3:00 p.m.). Serving sizes for protein are typically 3 ounces for women and 3 to 6 ounces for men. Limit red meat intake to a maximum of 12 ounces per week.

7. Soups should be low-sodium and broth-based, not cream-based; vegetable, bean, pea, and lentil soups are good options. Use Himalayan or Celtic sea salt instead of regular table salt (less than 1 teaspoon a day).

8. If organic foods are too expensive, choose organic for the foods you consume most often. If you can't buy organic, then choose very lean cuts of meat, peel the skin off poultry, thoroughly wash fruits and vegetables that cannot be peeled, and choose skim milk or 1 percent dairy products and skim milk cheese.

9. Avoid high-glycemic starches, including wheat and corn products, or at least decrease them dramatically. This includes all breads, crackers, bagels, potatoes, pasta, white rice, and corn. Avoid bananas and dried fruit.

10. Eat fresh, low-glycemic fruits only for breakfast or lunch and occasionally with morning and early afternoon snacks; eat steamed, stir-fried, or raw vegetables, lean meats, salads with colorful vegetables (preferably with a salad spritzer), raw nuts, and seeds.

11. Take fiber supplements such as two to four capsules of PGX fiber with 16 ounces of water before each meal and two to three PGX fiber capsules with each snack.

12. Do not eat later than 7:00 p.m.

APPENDIX B
RESOURCES AND SUPPLEMENTS

M OST OF THE products mentioned throughout this book are offered through Dr. Colbert's Divine Health Wellness Center or are available at your local health food store.

Divine Health Nutritional Products
  1908 Boothe Circle
  Longwood, FL 32750
  Phone: (407) 331-7007
  Web site: www.drcolbert.com
  E-mail: info@drcolbert.com

RESOURCES FOR WEIGHT LOSS
(From *The New Bible Cure for Weight Loss*)

Maintenance nutritional supplements
- Divine Health Active Multivitamin
- Divine Health Living Multivitamin
- Divine Health Green Supreme Food

Omega oils
- Divine Health Living Omega

Protein powders
- Divine Health Plant Protein
- Divine Health Living Protein

Supplements for weight loss
- Fat Loss Drops
- PGX fiber
- Living Green Tea with EGCG

- Living Green Coffee Bean
- Meratrim (Metabolic Lean)
- MBS 360: contains green coffee bean and green tea with EGCG and Irvingia (available at www.mbs360.tv) This contains three fat-burners in one pill.
- 7-keto-DHEA

Supplements for thyroid support
- Metabolic Advantage
- Iodine Synergy

To curb food cravings
- Serotonin Max
- N-acetyl-tyrosine
- 5-HTP

Supplements to boost energy
- Divine Health Adrenal Support
- Divine Health PQQ
- Cellgevity (supplement to quench inflammation)

NUTRITIONAL SUPPLEMENTS FOR DIABETES
(From *The New Bible Cure for Diabetes*)

Comprehensive multivitamin: Divine Health Multivitamin and Divine Health Living Multivitamin

Diabetic support: cinnulin, coffee berry, Divine Health Eye Sight, Divine Health Fiber, Divine Health Nutrients for Glucose Regulation, Irvingia, PGX fiber, pyridoxamine, Divine Health R Lipoic, Divine Health Vitamin D_3, and insulinase (cinnulin and chromium), benfotiamine, carnosine,

Omega Oils: Divine Health Omega Pure and Divine Health Living Omega

Metagenics
Alpha lipoic acid, 300 mg
(800) 692-9400 (refer to #W7741 when ordering)

www.drcolbert.meta-ehealth.com

WorldHealth.net

A global resource for antiaging medicine and to find a doctor that specializes in bioidentical hormone therapy

Life's Basics Protein

LifeTime Nutritional Specialties
www.lifetimevitamins.com/products/lifetime_plantprotein.html

ORDERING INFORMATION FOR SUPPLEMENTS

(From *The Bible Cure Recipes for Overcoming Candida*)

- Vaxa Buffer pH
  1-877-622-8292
  Provide #R.S. 49466

- Divine Health Candida Formula
  www.drcolbert.com

- Divine Health Probiotic
  www.drcolbert.com

- Moducare
  From most health food stores

- NAET
  To find a doctor in your area who performs NAET, visit their Web site at www.naet.com.

- Natur-Leaf
  1-888-532-7845

- Nystatin
  Call your physician or Pharmacy Specialists at 1-407-260-7002 to find a physician.

- Probiotic Pearls
  Integrative Therapeutics at 1-800-931-1709
  When prompted, provide Dr. Colbert's PCP #5266

- Total Leaky Gut by Nutri-West
  1-800-451-5620

- Three Lac
  1-760-542-3000
  Provide #ID 40274

- ALCAT
  This test must be performed by a physician.
  1-800-881-2685

- DSF
  Nutri-West
  1-800-451-5620

APPENDIX C
PASSPORT LIFE PROGRAM
(From *The Bible Cure Recipes for Overcoming Candida*)

ED McCLURE WEIGHED over 450 pounds before he was educated about candida and placed on the candida diet. Since implementing the diet and taking the required supplements, he has now lost over 200 pounds. This success filled Ed with a passion to help others suffering from candida. Ed and his wife, Elise, have developed The Passport Life Program in which he teaches seminars on how to overcome candida. For more information on this wonderful program, please visit their Web site at www.passportlife.com.

NOTES

(From *The New Bible Cure for Weight Loss*)

CHAPTER 1
YOU ARE GOD'S MASTERPIECE!

1. Centers for Disease Control and Prevention (CDC), "Overweight and Obesity: Defining Overweight and Obesity," http://www.cdc.gov/obesity /adult/defining.html (accessed March 19, 2013).
2. Centers for Disease Control and Prevention (CDC), "FastStats: Obesity and Overweight," http://www.cdc.gov/nchs/fastats/overwt.htm (accessed March 19, 2013).
3. Department of Health and Human Services, "Overweight and Obesity: Health Consequences," http://www.surgeongeneral.gov/library/calls /obesity/fact_consequences.html (accessed March 7, 2013).
4. Eric A. Finkelstein, Justin G. Trogdon, Joel W. Cohen, and William Dietz, "Annual Medical Spending Attributable to Obesity: Payer- and Service- Specific Estimates," *Health Affairs* 28, no. 5 (July 27, 2009): w822-w831; http://content.healthaffairs.org/content/28/5/w822.full.pdf+html (accessed March 7, 2013).

CHAPTER 2
DID YOU KNOW?—UNDERSTANDING OBESITY

1. Alicia G. Walton, "How Much Sugar Are Americans Eating [Infographic]," Forbes.com, August 30, 2012, http://www.forbes.com/sites/alicegwalton /2012/08/30/how-much-sugar-are-americans-eating-infographic/ (accessed March 7, 2013).
2. William Davis, *Wheat Belly* (New York: Rodale, 2011), 14.
3. H. C. Broeck, H. C. de Jong, E. M. Salentijn, et al., "Presence of Celiac Disease Epitopes in Modern and Old Hexaploid Wheat Varieties: Wheat Breeding May Have Contributed to Increased Prevalence of Celiac Disease," *Theoretical and Applied Genetics* 121, no. 8 (November 2010): 1527– 1539, as referenced in Davis, *Wheat Belly*, 26.
4. Davis, *Wheat Belly*, 35.
5. Ibid., 36. 53–54.
6. Ibid., 45.
7. Based on chart at BestDietTips.com, "Glycemic Index Food List (GI)," http://www.bestdiettips.com/glycemic-index-food-list-high-and-low-gi -index-foods-chart (accessed March 19, 2013).
8. Natalie Digate Muth, "Ask an Expert: What Are the Guidelines for Per- centage of Body Fat Loss?" The American Council on Exercise, December 2, 2009, http://www.acefitness.org/acefit/expert-insight-article/3/112/what -are-the-guidelines-for-percentage-of/ (accessed May 2, 2013).

CHAPTER 3
THE FOUNDATION OF HEALTHY EATING

1. US Department of Health and Human Services, *Dietary Guidelines for Americans, 2010*, 7th ed. (Washington DC: US Government Printing Office, 2010), 15; viewed at http://health.gov/dietaryguidelines/dga2010 /DietaryGuidelines2010.pdf (accessed March 20, 2013).
2. Kate Murphy, "The Dark Side of Soy," BusinessWeek.com, December 18, 2000, http://www.businessweek.com/2000/00_51/b3712218.htm (accessed September 17, 2009).

CHAPTER 4
POWER FOR CHANGE THROUGH DIET AND NUTRITION

1. MedicalNewsToday.com, "Mediterranean-Style Diet Reduces Cancer and Heart Disease Risk," June 26, 2003, http://www.medicalnewstoday.com /articles/3835.php (accessed March 20, 2013).
2. Antonia Trichopoulou, Pagona Lagiou, Hannah Kupeer, and Dimitrios Trichopoulos, "Cancer and the Mediterranean Dietary Traditions," *Cancer Epidemiology, Biomarkers and Prevention* 9 (September 2009): 869–873.
3. Gina Kolata, "Mediterranean Diet Shown to Ward Off Heart Attack and Stroke," New York Times, February 25, 2013, http://www.nytimes.com /2013/02/26/health/mediterranean-diet-can-cut-heart-disease-study-finds .html?pagewanted=all&_r=0 (accessed May 1, 2013).
4. Clara Felix, *All About Omega-3 Oils* (Garden City, NY: Avery Publishing, 1998), 32.
5. "Mercury Contamination in Fish: A Guide to Staying Healthy and Fighting Back," Natural Resources Defense Council, http://www.nrdc.org /health/effects/mercury/guide.asp (accessed May 1, 2013).
6. Robert Preidt, "Mom Was Right: Eating Soup Cuts Calorie Intake," May 1, 2007, ABCNews.com, http://abcnews.go.com/Health /Healthday/story?id=4506787&page=1 (accessed March 21, 2013).
7. Jennie Brand-Miller, Thomas M. S. Wolever, Kaye Foster-Powell, and Stephen Colagiuri, *The New Glucose Revolution*, 3rd ed., (New York: Marlow & Co., 2007), 86.
8. ScienceDaily.com, "Teens Who Eat Breakfast Daily Eat Healthier Diets Than Those Who Skip Breakfast," March 3, 2008, http://www.sciencedaily .com/releases/2008/03/080303072640.htm (accessed March 21, 2013).
9. K. N. Boutelle and D. S. Kirschenbaum, "Further Support for Consistent Self-Monitoring as a Vital Component of Successful Weight Control," *Obesity Research* 6, no. 3 (May 1998): 219–224, http://www.ncbi.nlm.nih .gov/pubmed/9618126 (accessed March 21, 2013).

CHAPTER 5
TIPS FOR EATING OUT

1. National Restaurant Association, "Restaurant Industry Sales Turn Positive in 2011 After Three Tough Years," RestaurantNews.com, February 1,

2011, http://www.restaurantnews.com/restaurant-industry-sales
-turn-positive-in-2011-after-three-tough-years/ (accessed March 26, 2013).

CHAPTER 6
POWER FOR CHANGE THROUGH ACTIVITY

1. Peter Jaret, "A Healthy Mix of Rest and Motion," *New York Times*, May 3, 2007, http://tinyurl.com/c7zxot3 (accessed March 26, 2013).
2. Centers for Disease Control and Prevention, "How Much Physical Activity Do Adults Need?", December 1, 2011, http://www.cdc.gov/physicalactivity /everyone/guidelines/adults.html (accessed March 26, 2013).

CHAPTER 7
SUPPLEMENTS THAT SUPPORT WEIGHT LOSS

1. LifeExtension.org, "Journal Abstracts: Green Coffee Bean Extract," *Life Extension Magazine*, February 2012, http://www.lef.org/magazine /mag2012/abstracts/feb2012_Green-Coffee-Bean-Extract_04.htm (accessed March 26, 2013).
2. Douglas Laboratories, "Metabolic Lean: Weight Management Formula," product data sheet, June 2012, http://www.douglaslabs.com/pdf/pds /201350.pdf (accessed March 26, 2013).
3. American Thyroid Association, "Iodine Deficiency," June 4, 2012, http:// www.thyroid.org/iodine-deficiency/ (accessed March 26, 2013).
4. J. A. Marlett, M. I. McBurney, J. L. Slavin, and American Dietetic Association, "Position of the American Dietetic Association: Health Implications of Dietary Fiber," *Journal of the American Dietetic Association* 102, no. 7 (2002): 993–1000.
5. N. C. Howarth, E. Saltzman, and S. B. Roberts, "Dietary Fiber and Weight Regulation," *Nutrition Review* 59, no. 5 (2001): 129–138.
6. Andrew Weil, "7-Keto: Supplement to Speed Metabolism?" DrWeil.com, http://www.drweil.com/drw/u/QAA401158/7Keto-Supplement-to-Speed -Metabolism.html (accessed May 2, 2013).
7. "7-Keto-DHEA," WebMD.com, http://www.webmd.com/vitamins -supplements/ingredientmono-835-7-KETO-DHEA.aspx?activeIngredient Id=835&activeIngredientName=7-KETO-DHEA (accessed May 2, 2013).
8. Weil, "7-Keto: Supplement to Speed Metabolism?"
9. J. L. Zenk, J. L. Frestedt, and M. A. Kuskowski, "HUM5007, a Novel Combination of Thermogenic Compounds, and 3-Acetyl-7-Oxo- Dehydroepiandrosterone: Each Increases the Resting Metabolic Rate of Overweight Adults," *Journal of Nutritional Biochemistry* 18, no. 9 (September 2007): 629–634; and Michael Davidson, Ashok Marwah, Ronald J. Sawchuk, et. al., "Safety and Pharmacokinetic Study With Escalating Doses of 3-Acetyl-7-Oxo-Dehydroepiandrosterone in Healthy Male volunteers," *Clinical Investigative Medicine* 23, no. 5 (October 2000): 300-310, abstract viewed at http://www.ncbi.nlm.nih.gov/pubmed/11055323 (accessed May 2, 2013).

10. Hoodia Advice, "The Science of Hoodia," http://www.hoodia-advice.org /hoodia-plant.html (accessed March 26, 2013).

11. Tom Mangold, "Sampling the Kalahari Hoodia Diet," BBC News, May 30, 2003, http://news.bbc.co.uk/2/hi/programmes/correspondent/2947810.stm (accessed March 26, 2013).

12. Ano Lobb, "Hepatoxicity Associated With Weight-Loss Supplements: A Case for Better Post-Marketing Surveillance, *World Journal of Gastroenterology* 15, no. 14 (April 14, 2009): 1786–1787, http://www.ncbi.nlm.nih.gov /pmc/articles/PMC2668789/ (accessed March 26, 2013).

13. Associated Press, "FDA Warns Consumers to Avoid Brazilian Diet Pills," USAToday.com, January 13, 2006, http://usatoday30.usatoday.com/news /health/2006-01-13-brazilian-diet-pills_x.htm (accessed March 26, 2013).

NOTES

(From *The New Bible Cure for Thyroid Disorders*)

CHAPTER 9
DO YOU HAVE A HIDDEN PROBLEM?

1. L. A. McKeown, "Everyone Over 35 Needs Thyroid Test, Group Says," WebMD Health, http://my.webmd.com/content/article/26/1728_58533 .htm (accessed November 23, 2003).
2. Richard Shames, M.D., and Karilee H. Shames, Ph.D., *Thyroid Power: Ten Steps to Total Health* (New York: HarperCollins, 2001), 2.

CHAPTER 10
A LAMP OF UNDERSTANDING

1. Mary Shoman, "Breaking News: Estrogen, Menopause and Thyroid," http://thyroid.about.com/library/weekly/aa042602a.htm (accessed November 23, 2003).
2. P. W. Ladenson, et al., "American Thyroid Association's Guidelines for Detection of Thyroid Dysfunction," *Arch Intern Med.* 160 (2000): 1573– 1575.
3. Elizabeth Smoots, M.D., FAAFP, "Is My Thyroid Overactive?", WebMD Health, http://my.webmd.com/content/article/42/1689_50865.htm? (accessed November 23, 2003).
4. The National Women's Health Information Center, "Graves' Disease," October 23, 2000, http://www.4woman.gov/faq/graves.htm (accessed November 23, 2003).
5. M. Sara Rosenthal, *The Thyroid Sourcebook* (Los Angeles: Lowell, 2000).
6. Ibid.

CHAPTER 11
FULL OF LIGHT—LIFESTYLE FACTORS

1. Glen Rothfeld, *Thyroid Balance* (Avon, MA: Adams Media, 2003).
2. Theo Colborn, et al., *Our Stolen Future* (New York: Plume Books, 1997), ii.
3. For more information on this topic, see www.perchlorateinfo.com.
4. David Kennedy, *Health Consciousness* 13 (3): 92–93.

CHAPTER 12
BRIGHTER AND BRIGHTER—SUPPLEMENTS

1. Joseph G. Hollowell, et al., "Iodine Nutrition in the United States. Trends and Public Health Implications: Iodine Excretion Data from National Health and Nutrition Examination Surveys I and III," *Journal of Clinical Endocrinology and Metabolism* 83 (10) (1998): 3401–3408.
2. For more information, see www.heartcenteronline.com.

3. Gonzzo Watson, D.C., "Adrenal Fatigue and a Holistic Approach to Recovery," http://www.watsonchiropractic.com/articles/adftg.htm (accessed November 24, 2003).

CHAPTER 13
A LIGHTED TEMPLE—NUTRITION

1. "Fighting Death, Disease, and Discomfort," NutritionStreet.com; http://www.nutitionstreet.com/fightingdisease.shtml: "The former Surgeon General of the United States, C. Everett Koop said of the 2.1 million deaths each year, 1.6 million (or 75 percent) were related to inadequate diet."

2. H. Roberts, *Aspartame Disease: An Ignored Epidemic* (N.p.: Sunshine Sentinel Press, 2001), 432.

NOTES

(From *The New Bible Cure for Diabetes*)

CHAPTER 15
A NEW BIBLE CURE WITH NEW HOPE FOR DIABETES

1. Diabetes Research Institute, "Diabetes Fact Sheet," http://www.diabetes research.org/Newsroom/DiabetesFactSheet (accessed July 28, 2009).
2. Centers for Disease Control and Prevention, "National Diabetes Fact Sheet," http://www.cdc.gov/diabetes/pubs/estimates.htm (accessed July 28, 2009).
3. World Health Organization, "What Is Diabetes?" http://www.who.int /mediacentre/factsheets/fs312/en/ (accessed July 28, 2009).
4. Centers for Disease Control and Prevention, "National Diabetes Fact Sheet."
5. Ibid.
6. Centers for Disease Control and Prevention, "Overweight Prevalence," http://www.cdc.gov/nchs/fastats/overwt.htm (accessed July 28, 2009).

CHAPTER 16
KNOW YOUR ENEMY

1. American Diabetes Association, "All About Diabetes," http://www.diabetes .org/about-diabetes.jsp (accessed July 28, 2009).
2. Ibid.
3. Centers for Disease Control and Prevention, "National Diabetes Fact Sheet."
4. American Diabetes Association, "A1C Test," http://www.diabetes.org/type -1-diabetes/a1c-test.jsp (accessed July 28, 2009).
5. Centers for Disease Control and Prevention, "National Diabetes Fact Sheet."
6. National Diabetes Information Clearinghouse, "National Diabetes Statistics, 2007," http://diabetes.niddk.nih.gov/dm/pubs/statistics/index .htm#complications (accessed July 28, 2009).
7. Centers for Disease Control and Prevention, "National Diabetes Fact Sheet."
8. The Diabetes Monitor, "Metabolic Syndrome," http://www.diabetes monitor.com/b429.htm (accessed July 29, 2009).
9. "Stress Treatments Helps Control Type 2 Diabetes," Mercola.com, http:// articles.mercola.com/sites/articles/archive/2002/01/23/stress-treatments.aspx (accessed July 29, 2009).
10. Ibid.
11. National Diabetes Data Group and National Institutes of Health, Diabetes in America, 2nd edition (Bethesda, MD: National Institutes of Health, 1995).

12. National Institute of Neurological Diseases and Stroke, "Transient Ischemic Attack Information Page," http://www.ninds.nih.gov/disorders/tia/tia.htm (accessed July 29, 2009).
13. Centers for Disease Control and Prevention, "National Diabetes Fact Sheet."
14. National Eye Institute, "Diabetic Retinopathy," http://www.nei.nih.gov/health/diabetic/retinopathy.asp (accessed July 29, 2009).
15. Centers for Disease Control and Prevention, "National Diabetes Fact Sheet."
16. Ibid.
17. Ibid.
18. Ibid.
19. Ibid.
20. Ibid.
21. Ibid.
22. "Erectile Dysfunction (Impotence) and Diabetes," WebMD.com, http://www.webmd.com/erectile-dysfunction/guide/ed-diabetes (accessed July 29, 2009).

CHAPTER 17
BATTLE DIABETES WITH GOOD NUTRITION

1. National Institutes of Health Office of Dietary Supplements, "Dietary Supplement Fact Sheet: Calcium," http://ods.od.nih.gov/factsheets/Calcium_pf.asp (accessed August 5, 2009).
2. Gabriel Cousens, There Is a Cure for Diabetes (Berkeley, CA: North Atlantic Books, 2008), 190–200.
3. Ibid., 179–182.
4. Dave Tuttle, "Controlling Blood Sugar With Cinnamon and Coffee Berry," Life Extension magazine, December 2005, as viewed online at http://www.lef.org/magazine/mag2005/dec2005_report_cinnamon_01.htm (accessed July 27, 2009).
5. Ibid.
6. Ibid.

CHAPTER 18
BATTLE DIABETES WITH ACTIVITY

1. Ming Wei, Larry W. Gibbons, Tedd L. Mitchell, James B. Kampert, Chong D. Lee, and Steven N. Blair, "The Association Between Cardiorespiratory Fitness and Impaired Fasting Glucose and Type 2 Diabetes Mellitus in Men," Annals of Internal Medicine, http://www.annals.org/cgi/content/abstract/130/2/89 (accessed July 29, 2009).
2. L. E. Davidson, R. Hudson, K. Kilpatrick, et al., "Effects of Exercise Modality on Insulin Resistance and Functional Limitation in Older Adults: a Randomized Controlled Trial," Archives of Internal Medicine 169, no. 2 (2009):122–131, as viewed online at http://archinte.ama-assn.org/cgi/content/abstract/169/2/122 on July 31, 2009.

CHAPTER 19
BATTLE DIABETES WITH WEIGHT LOSS

1. Centers for Disease Control and Prevention, "Defining Overweight and Obesity," http://www.cdc.gov/nccdphp/dnpa/obesity/defining.htm (accessed August 17, 2009).
2. Youfa Wang et al., "Comparison of Abdominal Adiposity and Overall Obesity in Predicting Risk of Type 2 Diabetes Among Men," American Journal of Clinical Nutrition 81, no. 3 (2005): 555–563.

CHAPTER 20
BATTLE DIABETES WITH NUTRIENTS AND SUPPLEMENTS

1. "Vitamin D Is the 'It' Nutrient of the Moment," ScienceDaily.com, http://www.sciencedaily.com/releases/2009/01/090112121821.htm (accessed July 30, 2009).
2. National Research Council, Food and Nutrition Board, Recommended Dietary Allowances, 10th edition (Washington DC: National Academy Press, 1989), as viewed online at http://ods.od.nih.gov/factsheets/chromium.asp#en17 (accessed July 27, 2009).
3. Neal D. Barnard, Dr. Neal Barnard's Program for Reversing Diabetes (New York: Rodale, 2007), 142.
4. National Institutes of Health Office of Dietary Supplements, "Dietary Supplement Fact Sheet: Chromium," http://ods.od.nih.gov/factsheets/chromium.asp (accessed July 27, 2009).
5. Richard Anderson, Noella Bryden, and Marilyn Polanski, "Chromium and Other Insuling Potentiators in the Prevention and Alleviation of Glucose Intolerance," United States Department of Agricultural Health, Agricultural Research Service, http://www.ars.usda.gov/research/publications/Publications.htm?seq_no_115=138818&pf=1 (accessed July 30, 2009).
6. Barnard, Dr. Neal Barnard's Program for Reversing Diabetes, 143.
7. Richard A. Anderson, "Chromium in the Prevention and Control of Diabetes," Diabetes and Metabolism (n.p., 2000), 22–27, as cited in Frank Murray, Natural Supplements for Diabetes (Laguna Beach, CA: Basic Health Publications, Inc. 2007), 114.
8. Ibid.
9. Richard A. Anderson, "Chromium, Glucose Intolerance and Diabetes" Journal of the American College of Nutrition 17, no. 6 (1998): 548–555, as viewed online at http://www.jacn.org/cgi/content/full/17/6/548 (accessed July 27, 2009).
10. Mark A. Mitchell, "Lipoic Acid: A Multitude of Metabolic Health Benefits," Life Extension magazine, October 2007, http://www.lef.org/LEFCMS/aspx/PrintVersionMagic.aspx?CmsID=115115 (accessed July 27, 2009).
11. John R. White, "Cinnamon: Should It Be Taken as a Diabetes Medication?" Diabetes Health, December 25, 2008. Accessed online at http://www.diabeteshealth.com/read/2008/12/25/5703/cinnamon-should-it-be-taken-as-a-diabetes-medication/ on July 27, 2009.

12. Mike Adams, "Study Shows Cinnulin Promotes Increase in Lean Body Mass and Reduction in Body Fat," NaturalNews.com, http://www.naturalnews.com/011852.html (accessed July 30, 2009).

13. Joslin Diabetes Center, "How Does Fiber Affect Blood Glucose Levels?" http://www.joslin.org/managing_your_diabetes_697.asp (accessed August 3, 2009).

14. James W. Anderson, Dr. Anderson's High-Fiber Fitness Plan (Lexington, KY: University Press of Kentucky, 1994), 14.

15. Michael Murray, "What Makes People Fat, Why Diets Don't Work, and What Triggers Appetite?" SmartBomb.com, http://www.smartbomb.com/drmurrayweight.html (accessed July 30, 2009).

16. "Good Bye to Fad Diets, Revolutionary Natural Fibre Discovered in Canada," MedicalNewsToday.com, http://www.medicalnewstoday.com/articles/12058.php (accessed July 30, 2009).

17. PGX, "Frequently Asked Questions," www.pgx.com/us/en/faq (accessed July 27, 2009).

18. Chris Lydon, "Turn Off Your Fat Switch: Understanding the Risks of Leptin Resistance," Life Extension magazine (April/May/June 2009), 49–55.

19. Ibid.

20. "Trans Fat, NOT Saturated Fat, Increases Diabetes," American Journal of Nutrition 73, (June 2001): 1001–1002, 1019–1026, as viewed at http://articles.mercola.com/sites/articles/archive/2001/06/16/diabetes-part-four.aspx (accessed August 3, 2009).

21. Laurie Barclay, "Unique Form of Vitamin B6 Protects Against Complications Related to Diabetes and Aging," Life Extension magazine, October 2008, as viewed online at http://www.lef.org/magazine/mag2008/oct2008_Vitamin-B6-Protects-Against-Diabetes-Aging_02.htm (accessed July 31, 2009).

22. Julius G. Goepp, "Protecting Against Glycation and High Blood Sugar With Benfotiamine," Life Extension magazine, April 2008, as viewed online at http://search.lef.org/cgi-src-bin/MsmGo.exe?grab_id=0&page_id=919&query=benfotiamine&hiword=BENFOTIAMIN%20BENFOTIAMINES%20benfotiamine%20 (accessed July 31, 2009).

23. U. S. Department of Health and Human Services, "Polycystic Ovary Syndrome (PCOS)," WomensHealth.gov, http://www.womenshealth.gov/faq/polycystic-ovary-syndrome.cfm (accessed July 31, 2009).

NOTES

(From *The Bible Cure for Candida and Yeast Infections*)

CHAPTER 23
GET INFORMED

1. Michael Colgan, *The New Nutrition* (San Diego: C. I. Publications, 1994).
2. William G. Crook, *The Yeast Connection Handbook* (Jackson, TN: Professional Books, 1999), 15–19.
3. Adapted from Crook, *The Yeast Connection Handbook*, 15–19.

CHAPTER 24
RESTORE YOUR HEALTH WITH NUTRITION

1. For more information on the glycemic index, see the glycemic index chart in *The Bible Cure for Weight Loss and Muscle Gain*, 12–15.

CHAPTER 27
RECHARGE YOUR SPIRIT WITH FAITH

1. Norman Cousins, *Anatomy of an Illness As Perceived by the Patient* (Norton, NY: Bantam, 1979).
2. S. I. McMillen, *None of These Diseases* (Westwood, NJ: Revell, 1963), 7.

NOTES

(From *The Bible Cure Recipes for Overcoming Candida*)

CHAPTER 30
LAYING THE GROUND RULES

1. Adapted from William G. Crook, *The Yeast Connection Handbook* (Jackson, TN: Professional Books, 1999), 15–19.

CHAPTER 31
YUMMY BREAKFASTS

1. Gail Burton, *The Candida Control Cookbook* (Fairfield, CT: Aslan Publishing, 1995), 59.
2. Ed and Elisa McClure, *Eat Your Way to Heal-Thy Life* (Boerne, TX: Passport Life Center), 92. Ed and Lisa are founders of Passport Life Center. Visit their Web site at www.passportlife.com. Used by permission.
3. Ibid., 93.
4. Ibid., 95.
5. Ibid., page not given.
6. Ibid.

CHAPTER 32
SIMPLE SALADS

1. Crook, *The Yeast Connection Handbook*, 222.
2. McClure, *Eat Your Way to Heal-Thy Life*.
3. Ibid., 44.
4. Ibid., 35.
5. Ibid., 38.
6. Ibid., 45.
7. Ibid., page not given.
8. Ibid., 41.
9. Burton, *The Candida Control Cookbook*, 144.
10. Ibid.
11. Ibid., 145.

CHAPTER 33
ENTICING ENTRÉES

1. Burton, *The Candida Control Cookbook*, 82.
2. Ibid., 85.
3. McClure, *Eat Your Way to Heal-Thy Life*.
4. Ibid.
5. Burton, *The Candida Control Cookbook*, 91.
6. McClure, *Eat Your Way to Heal-Thy Life*, 62.
7. Burton, *The Candida Control Cookbook*, 72.
8. Ibid., 69.

9. Karen Tripp, *Candida Recipe Collection*, as viewed at http://www.geocities .com/HotSprings/4966/marinade.htm.
10. Burton, *The Candida Control Cookbook*, 103.
11. McClure, *Eat Your Way to Heal-Thy Life*.
12. Ibid., 46.
13. Ibid., 47.
14. Ibid., 50.
15. Ibid., 52.
16. Ibid., 53.

CHAPTER 34
VIRTUOUS VEGETABLES

1. Burton, *The Candida Control Cookbook*, 110.
2. McClure, *Eat Your Way to Heal-Thy Life*.
3. Burton, *The Candida Control Cookbook*, 112.
4. McClure, *Eat Your Way to Heal-Thy Life*, 75.
5. Ibid., 73.
6. Ibid., 72.
7. Ibid., page not given.
8. Burton, *The Candida Control Cookbook*, 119.
9. Ibid., 125.

CHAPTER 35
DELICIOUS DESSERTS

1. Tripp, Candida Recipe Collection as viewed at http://www.geocities.com /HotSprings/4966/tapioca.htm.
2. Burton, *The Candida Control Cookbook*, 152.
3. McClure, *Eat Your Way to Heal-Thy Life*, 85.
4. Ibid., 86.
5. Ibid., 87.
6. Burton, *The Candida Control Cookbook*, 186.
7. Ibid., 187.
8. Ibid., 189.

CHAPTER 36
SCRUMPTIOUS SOUPS, SNACKS AND APPETIZERS

1. Burton, *The Candida Control Cookbook*, 54.
2. McClure, *Eat Your Way to Heal-Thy Life*, 32.
3. Ibid., 33.
4. *Candida Albicans Yeast-Free Cookbook*, 63.
5. McClure, *Eat Your Way to Heal-Thy Life*, 30.
6. Ibid., 16.
7. Ibid., 17.
8. Ibid.
9. Ibid., 18.
10. Ibid., 19

CHAPTER 37
AND THAT'S NOT ALL!

1. McClure, *Eat Your Way to Heal-Thy Life*, 21.
2. Burton, *The Candida Control Cookbook*, 38.
3. Ibid., 40.
4. McClure, *Eat Your Way to Heal-Thy Life*, 25.
5. Ibid., 29.
6. Ibid., page not given.
7. Ibid.
8. Karen Tripp in Chyrel's Kitchen as viewed at http://www/linkline.com /personal/gingen/season/chilifre.htm.
9. Ibid., as viewed at http://www/linkline.com/personal/gingen/season/creole2 .htm.
10. Burton, *The Candida Control Cookbook*, 37.

A PERSONAL NOTE

From Don Colbert

G OD DESIRES TO heal you of disease. His Word is full of promises that confirm His love for you and His desire to give you His abundant life. His desire includes more than physical health for you; He wants to make you whole in your mind and spirit as well as through a personal relationship with His Son, Jesus Christ.

If you haven't met my best friend, Jesus, I would like to take this opportunity to introduce Him to you. It is very simple. If you are ready to let Him come into your life and become your best friend, all you need to do is sincerely pray this prayer:

> *Lord Jesus, I want to know You as my Savior and Lord. I believe You are the Son of God and that You died for my sins. I also believe You were raised from the dead and now sit at the right hand of the Father praying for me. I ask You to forgive me for my sins and change my heart so that I can be Your child and live with You eternally. Thank You for Your peace. Help me to walk with You so that I can begin to know You as my best friend and my Lord. Amen.*

If you have prayed this prayer, you have just made the most important decision of your life. I rejoice with you in your decision and your new relationship with Jesus. Please contact my publisher at pray4me@charismamedia.com so that we can send you some materials that will help you become established in your relationship with the Lord. We look forward to hearing from you.

ABOUT THE AUTHOR

DON COLBERT, MD, was born in Tupelo, Mississippi. He attended Oral Roberts School of Medicine in Tulsa, Oklahoma, where he received a bachelor of science degree in biology in addition to his degree in medicine. Dr. Colbert completed his internship and residency with Florida Hospital in Orlando, Florida. He is board certified in family practice and anti-aging medicine and has received extensive training in nutritional medicine.

If you would like more information about natural and divine healing, or information about *Divine Health nutritional products*, you may contact Dr. Colbert at:

Don Colbert, MD
1908 Boothe Circle
Longwood, FL 32750
Telephone: 407-331-7007 (for ordering products only)
Website: www.drcolbert.com.

Disclaimer: Dr. Colbert and the staff of Divine Health Wellness Center are prohibited from addressing a patient's medical condition by phone, facsimile, or e-mail. Please refer questions related to your medical condition to your own primary care physician.

PICK UP THESE OTHER
GREAT BIBLE CURE BOOKS

by Don Colbert, MD:

The Bible Cure for ADD and Hyperactivity
The Bible Cure for Allergies
The Bible Cure for Arthritis
The Bible Cure for Asthma
The Bible Cure for Autoimmune Diseases
The Bible Cure for Back Pain
The Bible Cure for Colds, Flu, and Sinus Infections
The Bible Cure for Headaches
The Bible Cure for Heartburn and Indigestion
The Bible Cure for Hepatitis and Hepatitis C
The Bible Cure for High Cholesterol
The Bible Cure for Irritable Bowel Syndrome
The Bible Cure for Memory Loss
The Bible Cure for Menopause
The Bible Cure for PMS and Mood Swings
The Bible Cure for Prostate Disorders
The Bible Cure for Skin Disorders
The New Bible Cure for Cancer
The New Bible Cure for Chronic Fatigue and Fibromyalgia
The New Bible Cure for Depression and Anxiety
The New Bible Cure for Heart Disease
The New Bible Cure for High Blood Pressure
The New Bible Cure for Osteoporosis
The New Bible Cure for Sleep Disorders
The New Bible Cure for Stress